Weight Loss For People In A Hurry

How to lose the most amount of weight,

in the least amount of time,

and keep it off.

By Sam Van Horn

Table of Contents

Introduction

A Fork In The Road

At some point we come to a fork in the road. One leads to triggered weight gain and the other leads to a lean healthy life. The illusion is that it is a conscious decision to make.

What if there was a "fat trigger"? This would be a biological mechanism that caused you to gain weight, seek out fattening foods, and turn off your natural fat burning hormones. If there was such a trigger then our weight loss strategy would be simple, stop triggering weight gain. The only way to find something like that would be to observe it in nature, across multiple species that gain weight seasonally, and see if there is a common mechanism. So that is exactly what they did. Researchers have observed animals that gain weight before prolonged periods of starvation and have identified one process, caused by one nutrient, in one organ that makes their whole metabolism go off the rails. If you have any fat on your belly you've triggered this same mechanism.

This manual will walk you through identifying the exact trigger for weight gain and then teach you how to melt your excess fat away in the shortest possible time.

Who Is This Program For?

This program is for beginners. For sure there are benefits for seasoned weight loss veterans that have tried and failed every other eating plan on the market but at the end of the day, the less cluttered your mind is, the better. Sometimes, people who have been around a particular subject for awhile tend to filter out the parts they don't want to hear, this is especially true for serial dieters.

Start with the goal in mind. This program is specifically designed to help you lose weight. For sure there are other nutritional goals that are important (longevity, gut health, etc.) and those goals may call for a different strategy but for right now let's just focus on jump starting your weight loss. It is my hope that you use this manual as a launch pad to continually investigate and upgrade you and your family's personal diet and lifestyle to be free from preventable disease. To this end, I am going to introduce you to some science that can change the way you look and feel.

The weight loss you experience is essentially the bait intended to draw you into a rabbit hole of learning about your health, constantly upgrading your diet, and turn you into your own researcher (or you could just lose the weight if you want to).

This program is dedicated to helping people achieve weight loss, ALL people. Even those who happen to be on a very strict budget. Poverty and obesity go hand-in-hand. Obesity is far more prevalent in lower income neighborhoods. The low cost of sugar, corn syrup, and wheat are just as tempting as the treats themselves. Have you ever been to a dollar store? The aisles in discount stores are lined with refined sugar, high fructose corn syrup, and wheat. These are by far the cheapest ingredients because they are subsidized by our own government. Our government is effectively subsidizing the obesity epidemic.[1] I created this program with these restrictions in mind. I will tell you to eat cheap vegetables if that's all you can afford or have time for. You can still follow the program with more expensive, organic, non-GMO foods but try not to be a dick about it. Being healthy is a basic human right, it shouldn't be cost or time prohibitive and it shouldn't involve social shame.

What Success Looks Like

You're likely reading this book because of the promise on the cover, if that's the case you will not be disappointed. In the third week of this program you will lose weight faster than you ever have before and because of the hormonal adaptations, it will stay off.

Our first goal is quick fat loss (almost every diet can do this). Our second and more important goal is to change your internal environment to make it harder for you to gain the weight back (almost no diet can do this). It can be done, we all know someone who will stay lean no matter how much they eat, you can mimic a similar environment in your own body over time. We just need to change how your body reacts to food. As you'll soon see it all comes down to satiety hormones, insulin sensitivity, and insulin resistance.

---

[1] http://time.com/4393109/food-subsidies-obesity/

About Me

First of all, I am just as dumb as you are. Some of the terms and mechanism is this manual took me a long time to understand. As long as we don't get scared away by crazy long words we will be fine, the more you see them the better you will understand them. Don't worry about seeing a new term or not understanding something, I will break it down for people like us.

I am just smart enough to find people smarter than me and tell you what I learned. In my first biology lecture from Massachusetts Institute of Technology's Dr. Eric Lander, he mentioned that we would be learning new material that was previously unavailable to biology students. You see, our collective knowledge about the human body advances faster than any other technical innovation, including Moore's law (Moore's law is the reason you need a new iPhone every 18 months). It's because of this ever expanding feature of biology that this has to be a continuously evolving strategy. If you know that I am wrong about something, show me the evidence and I will humbly correct it. You can and should help refine this program.

I've studied biology, endocrinology and, to a lesser extent, behavioral psychology through mostly audit courses. My days consist of listen to lectures, podcasts, audio books, and interviews. Once I have a grasp on the vernacular of a given field I prefer podcasts and interviews to courses simply because podcasts give you the most up-to-date information. Any given concept in biology can change directions drastically over just a few weeks.

Some of the concepts in this manual have been around since the dawn of medicine but we are only recently uncovering what specifically make them work (i.e. autophagy). I'm sure, between the time I type this and the time you read this, there will be a ton of new insights about these mechanisms. This is what fascinates me the most: I never have to stop learning and communicating these biological concepts.

I am hoping to get this information in your hands so it can be useful to you and your family before you experience any sadness or loss because of obesity or any of the other metabolic diseases.

You see, my Mother died in my arms four years ago from lung cancer. At the time I knew next to nothing about the disease, jump ahead a few months, a few text books, and a few lectures later and I could, at the very least, have had a decent if not skeptical conversation about her therapy with her Doctors.

Last year, on November 29th my Father succumbed to his decades long battle with type II diabetes. One of his biggest fears, after a scare in the late 90's was losing his leg to the disease. So it seems a little...unfair...that they amputated his leg three days before he died. Again, after the fact, I know pretty much everything I could know about the disease without a formal education.

Could I have saved either one of my parents? Probably not. They were in their 70's and I feel like they were dying for the last couple of decades. What I could do and what I set my mind to accomplish, was to make damn sure that my two daughters (Josephine 9 & Penelope 7) never experience the helplessness I felt watching my Mom & Dad melt away.

I seemed to always be reacting instead of preventing. This manual is my attempt to prevent metabolic disease in my friends and family and by extension your friends and family.

So, aside from personal tragedy, I've basically been in the restaurant business for half of my life (I've opened over a dozen restaurants). I am also a NASM CPT. I have hundreds of clients across the globe whom I coach through an online eating group. I've written a ton of different niche specific manuals from building businesses to losing weight. I essentially like to simplify and communicate complicated systems in a way that children could explain them back to me.

Plus, when I turned 40, I was fat, sick, unhealthy, and depressed. Now at 44, I have muscles, abs, and energy (I understand what it takes to fix it). For the last four years I have worked closely with hundreds of people to help them lose thousands of pounds, this is ultimately what led to this program.

Medical disclaimer/ Terms of use

(1) No advice

This manual contains general information about medical conditions, nutrition, health, and diets. The information is not advice and should not be treated as such.

(2) No warranties

The medical information in this manual is provided without any representations or warranties, expressed or implied. We make no representations or warranties in relation to the medical information found in this this manual.

Before starting any diet, you should speak to your doctor. You must not rely on the information in this manual as an alternative to medical advice from your doctor or other professional healthcare provider. If you have any specific questions about any medical matter, you should consult your doctor or other professional healthcare provider first.

If you think you may be suffering from any medical condition, you should seek immediate medical attention. You should never delay seeking medical advice, disregard medical advice, or discontinue medical treatment because of information in this manual.

These are the terms of use for this manual. If you do not accept these terms of use, please do not use this manual. Your continued use of this manual confirms your acceptance of these terms.

Section 1: The Science and Biology of Weight Loss

In this section we will lay the foundation of exactly how the body works when it comes to losing weight. When you take the time to understand the mechanism you can troubleshoot your own weight loss and tweak your strategy when necessary.

How To Science

Dogma: "a belief or set of beliefs that is accepted by the members of a group without being questioned or doubted". You see dogma in just about every area of life. You have dogmatic religious folk, crossfit people, paleo practitioners, low carb advocates, personal trainers, and vegans. The problem is you also have dogmatic clinicians and dogmatic scientists. When a central belief is unquestioned you run the risk of every decision made on the basis of that belief spiralling way off course. This is extremely dangerous when it comes to our health.

Here are some examples of dogmatic principles for weight loss gone wrong:
> "A calorie is a calorie"
> "Eat less and move more to lose weight"
> "Saturated fat causes heart disease"
> "Meat causes cancer"
> "If you do not eat you will go into starvation mode, hold onto fat, and burn muscle"

These belong right up there with:
> "The earth is flat"
> "If she floats, she's a Witch"
> "The leeches will suck the poison out"

All of these opinions have shaped the way we think about certain topics and they are simply not true. When it comes to you and your family's health, question everything.

Facts and evidence are all that matter. If you don't understand or trust the scientific method, what can make you change your mind? If you understand science, new evidence can change your mind. If you don't understand science then you may be stuck with your conclusions whether they are right or wrong.

When we hear a claim we need to look for references to non-biased, independently funded, peer-reviewed studies in established medical or science journals.

If you just use a standard search engine you will get the most popular results not the most accurate results. The problem is that most of us just want our ideology confirmed so we will type in biased phrases like "how do GMO's kill people" then read the most popular blog posts in a never ending, biased, positive feedback loop, often with zero references.

When you learn to read published science or medical journals you don't have to take anyone's word as fact, and you shouldn't. What you should do is look for published scientific papers if it sounds improbable. If someone makes a claim and doesn't have solid published references ("Guru" blog posts don't count) then you should probably ignore it. If some advice sounds fishy, check Google scholar, PubMed, and/ or Medline.

Pubmed is the go-to site for professional researchers, clinicians, and other nerds. Google scholar references published medical/ science journals and universities while filtering out "natural news" sites and scam artists trying to profit from everyone's fear and ignorance (like David Wolfe, Gwyneth Paltrow, Food Babe, etc.) and Medline references over 26 million published/ reviewed medical papers.

If you want to learn more about how to distinguish fact from bullshit there is a fantastic book on the subject of bad research called "Bad Science: Quacks, Hacks, and Big Pharma Flacks" by Ben Goldacre.

About You

You are a precious snowflake! You have unique genetic polymorphisms (your genes are different than other people's genes) that will make your body and brain respond to food in dramatically different ways than the person sitting next to you. This is also a reason why some diets just won't work for you. It's up to you to test and tweak everything.

For instance, when it comes to blood glucose response (how your body reacts to sugar) yours could go crazy just by eating a banana but have zero response to eating a cookie, while your friend can reach prediabetic levels of blood sugar with that same cookie.[2] These genetic variants make it impossible to have a perfect diet that everyone should follow. This is likely due to where your ancestors spent their time and for which foods they've developed tolerances and intolerances.

Although your genes can overreact to certain foods, the idea that this is why you've gained weight just doesn't hold up under scrutiny. In 1900, only about 3% of the population of the United States was considered obese, compare that to more than 30% today! Genetics can only account for a small amount of your weight gain, you or your parents are likely the fattest people in your entire ancestry. If you are obese, how deep into your family history would you have to go to find someone that wasn't considered obese? Probably only 2 or 3 generations. Your Great Grandmother was most likely very lean, along with her entire generation and every generation before her.

With individual genetic variations in mind there are still some universal truths that can apply to broad sections of most populations. The following is true for everyone no matter where their ancestors are from:
1. Vegetable fiber is absolutely necessary for gut health.
2. Going long periods without food (fasting) is crucial for your body's natural repair processes (autophagy).
3. Eating dietary fat is essential for your body to function properly.
4. Refined sugar, corn, and wheat are really bad for you.

Those are the tenets that are applicable to almost everyone. If you want to figure out what your specific genes mean for you, you can go to 23andme.com, get their basic report, then plug it into promethease.com and discuss it with your doctor.

---

[2] https://wis-wander.weizmann.ac.il/life-sciences/blood-sugar-levels-response-foods-are-highly-individual

It's All Relative

Another reason, besides genetics, that there are no one-size-fits-all diets is that we are all starting from different places. If you eat twenty Snickers bars everyday then you suddenly cut down to ten bars a day, you are going to lose weight. You might even write a book telling people to start eating ten candy bars every day to lose weight! On the other hand, If you usually only eat five Snickers per day and you crank it up a notch to ten, you are going to start gaining weight pretty quickly.

Similarly, how your Mom ate when she was pregnant with you has likely modified your internal environment. If your Mom was diagnosed with hypothyroidism you would have increased beta cell proliferation in your pancreas (causing more insulin secretion) and if your Mother was diagnosed with gestational diabetes, you are going to overproduce insulin as a baby leading to fetal macrosomia (being a big fat baby). These are not life sentences though, you can break the cycle of fat mom, fat baby, fat mom. This manual will be a good start, getting your doctor involved will boost your likelihood of success.

Where you start will determine the speed of your weight loss and might cause you to modify your strategy.

You Are Not A Food Scientist

Nutritionism is a termed coined by Author Michael Pollan in his book "In Defense of Food". It is an ideology that maintains that the value of food is in it's nutrients and not in the food itself. In other words, food is seen as a delivery system for nutrients – rather than as a whole. Carbohydrates, lipids, fibers, amino acids, proteins and calories are broad terms for giant categories.

Using a biochemist's vernacular is one way us personal trainers make you think we are smarter than you (we are not). Broccoli, kale, cookies, and maple syrup are all carbohydrates but they all have very different effects on your hormones. For anyone to tell you to eat any number of carbs is simplifying instructions beyond the point of usefulness. In this manual we'll stay away from calling foods by their categories and just call them by their names.

While we're at it, using any sort of math in your diet is just confusing and unnecessary if you're not a physique model or a professional athlete.

Why Most Diets Can Work

No matter what weight loss plan you choose to follow they will all start to work for just one reason: You will eat and drink less sugar than you used to. Which means you are not spiking your insulin hormone as much as before.

Insulin is a hormone that comes out when you eat to clear your blood of sugar (glucose). Known as the "storage" hormone, insulin puts glucose in your liver, your muscles and your body fat. With insulin present you cannot lose body fat. If your insulin is constantly spiked your cells become insulin resistant over time. When your cells refuse to respond to insulin your pancreas releases more insulin, your body then starts to create new fat cells (de novo lipogenesis) and if you don't stop spiking your insulin every day those cells become insulin resistant too! This is the beginning of type II diabetes and it can kill you. Insulin turns off fat burning and turns on fat storing.

Every single person who has had success with any diet has spiked their insulin less than they used to. When people start a diet they eliminate the most obvious offenders: Soda, alcohol, ice cream, french fries, cake, etc. and this leads to their early successes. This strategy is incomplete though, as it does not address the actual reason those foods make us fat in the first place. We will get to that.

Why Most Diets Stop Working

There are three major reasons why most diets fail.
1. Homeostasis and resting metabolic rate (RMR). Homeostasis is your body's way of staying the same. When you get hot your body tries to cool itself by sweating, when you get cold your body tries to heat itself by shivering. Homeostasis is your body's built in thermostat for everything. If you gain a few pounds your body will try to lose them, if you lose a few pounds the body will try to get them back.

Your body will always try to get back to a set body weight, it will manipulate your resting metabolic rate (RMR) to do this. Your resting metabolic rate (RMR) is the amount of energy you are constantly using without exercise. Depending on how you lose weight this can go up or down. We want it to go up. We need to change our body's set point (RMR) to accommodate a lower body fat percentage. Essentially, as we lose weight with this program, we are telling our body "this is who we are now", our hormones will fight to keep us at this new weight. Once we do that it will be difficult to gain the weight back.

2. Insulin resistance. We can lose a ton of weight but if we don't change how our bodies react (or overreact) to food we will plateau and our bodies will try really hard to gain the weight back because of homeostasis. We absolutely have to return to an insulin sensitive state if we want any lasting changes. You cannot change your body's set point, and RMR, without manipulating your insulin sensitivity.

3. Convenience. Probably THE biggest reason people stop their diets is the sheer inconvenience of it! I'm telling you right now that you cannot keep up a disruptive routine for very long. Your new routine has to be at least as easy as your old routine or you're wasting your time.

The strategies in the program will address any form of inconvenience that may come up. You do not have to become a nutritional expert, count calories, weigh your food, meal prep every Sunday, or stop eating at fast food places, you don't even have to learn how to cook to lose weight! You can eat in your car. You can microwave stuff. In fact, if it's not convenient, you will have an incredibly hard time sticking to it.

Calories?

The prevailing theory is that we eat too much and move too little. It is "calories in versus calories out" according to politicians, clinicians, soda companies, most personal trainers, anyone selling candy, anyone selling diet food, anyone selling exercise products, and just about everyone you will ever ask about weight gain. The problem is, it's just not true.

Calories in versus calories out, otherwise know as the "energy balance theory", relies on the first law of thermodynamics. This law requires a closed system (not affected by outside forces) which the human body certainly is not. We assume that calories-in is totally independent of calories-expended, we are wrong. If we ate a little less and our calories-out stayed the same then this strategy would work great! But, the body doesn't work like that. If you eat less the body will compensate by downregulating some of its internal processes like hair growth, bone growth, body temperature, heart beat, blood pressure and volume, etc. to compensate.[3] After all, most of our calories out have nothing to do with exercise or movement.

---

[3] https://www.ncbi.nlm.nih.gov/pubmed/2204100

This theory also assumes that all calories, no matter the source, have the exact same effect on the body, they don't. If you eat 1,000 calories of cookies you will have a flood of insulin and dopamine then finally a spike in ghrelin. These are all hormones related to appetite signalling and fat storage. This combination of hormones will lead to spikes and crashes every few hours. If you eat 1,000 calories of steak you will get a smaller rise in these same hormones but spread out over time, not the giant spikes we were never exposed to until the last few decades. With the steak you will also get a rise in satiety hormones (peptide YY, cholecystokinin, etc.) that tell you to stop eating. You'll also get proteins to build and repair your body and saturated fats which are absolutely necessary for the body. None of the calories from the cookies are necessary.

The bottom line is this: If you have two identical people, consuming identical calories, can you make one fatter or thinner than the other without changing the amount of calories they eat or use? The answer is a resounding yes.

So why does this strategy seem to work for some people? The "move more, eat less" strategy can work if what you're eating less of is refined sugar and wheat. We run into problems with this strategy when we also eat less of the foods that contribute to feeling full and we "move" enough to make us hungry. Over time this strategy will backfire which is why you will never see a "Biggest Loser" reunion show, almost all of the contestants have gained the weight back and then some! Their resting metabolic rate (metabolism) drops incredibly low to accommodate the decrease in calories causing the inevitable weight regain.[4]

Physique competitors need to monitor every aspect of their diets, especially in those crucial few weeks before competition. All of their food is pre planned and now they must titrate down to an exact amount (using calories), they have no intention of eating to satiety. This is the population that can benefit from counting calories. They have an entirely different (although extremely temporary) environment than most of us and are well aware of their body's hormonal response to the food they've chosen. What do you think happens to their weight and body fat percentage in the days following a competition?

Calories should still remain the benchmark for measuring food energy if you are following a diet that has already addressed the hormonal effects of refined sugar and wheat. For instance, a ketogenic diet demands that seventy to ninety percent of your diet consist of fat. The only way to get this number would be to break your entire diet down into calories. Despite this, the fact remains that simply reducing calories on a high sugar diet, will not lead to lasting weight loss.

---

[4] https://www.ncbi.nlm.nih.gov/pubmed/27136388

If you observe someone lose weight you might see a drop in their calories. If you see someone gain weight you might see an increase in their calories. Or you may see the opposite. The amount of calories only correlates (happens at the same time) with fluctuations in body weight, it does not cause any long term changes so it cannot be the cure. For this program you will see calories as more of a correlation rather than a cause of success. We won't bother measuring them.

So, if it's not calories, what is causing obesity? Ask yourself this: does a baby grow because he's eating too much or is he eating too much because he is growing? A baby's biological weight gain is triggered at conception and remains on until early adulthood, then it switches off. If you're getting fat, you've triggered fat gain. You're not getting fat because you're eating too much, you're eating too much because you're getting fat. Your body is storing fat and sugar while creating new fat cells because it is stressed or damaged.

It works like this:
1. Your body gets triggered into storage mode
2. You seek out foods that will fatten you up
3. You expend less energy

In response to a biological trigger there are storage factors reacting to this stress that will make you eat and you can't stop them once they are signalled, even if you eat less. If you do "eat less" food you will "use less" energy for basic functions in favor of storage. What you can do is stop signalling storage hormones and start repairing the damage. The damage that I'm talking about is hepatic (liver related) insulin resistance leading to chronically high insulin levels (hyperinsulinemia). There are also damaged mitochondria that will not metabolize fat properly because of sugar consumption.

Mitochondria are the power plants of the cell that turn fat and/ or glucose into energy. In a healthy cell the mitochondria are always burning body fat. If you eat a bunch of sugar they can easily switch over and use that sugar and return to normal when the sugar is used up, this is called metabolic flexibility. Your mitochondria can become damaged and defective if they are constantly burning sugar, or you have a buildup of uric acid, and are never allowed to dip into the cell's fat stores. When your mitochondria use glucose they are making fat, when they are making fat, they will not burn fat. Insulin prevents your mitochondria from burning fat, constant insulin will constantly stop your mitochondria from burning fat.

Obesity comes down to a molecular trigger followed by physical cellular damage, hormonal signalling, tolerance and resistance. All of these are directly affected over time by a steady diet of refined sugar and wheat. With this in mind you can envision what food labels should actually say. Each label should list the short and long term effects on your body versus a bunch of arbitrary percentages.

Hormones

How your body makes you make decisions. Have you ever wanted to sleep or not sleep, eat or not eat, have sex, or even just punch somebody in the face. These behaviors, just as every other behavior, are all controlled by your hormones. You can fight against them but you will eventually lose, however, you can manipulate some of them. You can calm yourself down with some deep breathing, you can make yourself tired with exercise, and you can absolutely turn on your "stop eating" hormones by changing which foods you eat.

A hormone is any member of a class of signaling molecules produced by glands in multicellular organisms that are transported by the circulatory system to target distant organs to regulate physiology and behaviour.

Your entire body is tightly regulated by which hormones are present. Your energy metabolism and fat accumulation are no exceptions. If you are going to grow or if you are going to shrink you will need to activate the corresponding hormones. There are prescription drugs that will cause you to get fat by manipulating your hormones and it will not matter what your calories are, how much willpower you have, or whether your parents were lean or not.

Can You Get Fat Without Changing Your Diet?

I want to highlight this section just to show you evidence that weight gain and fat accumulation is not a simple matter of calories in versus calories out (energy balance theory). Instead, we need to understand that weight gain, once triggered, is absolutely influenced by the hormonal effects of foods and stress (hormonal theory).

You can get fat without any dietary changes if you change your hormonal environment to favor obesity. For example, when prescribed insulin or insulin raising drugs (Sulfonylureas, Amylin mimetics, Glinides, etc.) people gain weight in a dose dependent manner. When patients are prescribed a lot of insulin, patients gain a lot of weight. When patients are prescribed a little insulin, patients gain a little weight. When prescribed Insulin lowering drugs (Metformin) patients lost weight. This happens in everyone regardless of calories, exercise, genetics, or willpower.

Most of us are born with insulin sensitivity. Most of us wake up every morning in an insulin sensitive state. This morning rhythm will stay this way until we break our metabolism and become resistant to insulin.

In an insulin sensitive environment it works like this: we eat a little sugar, the pancreas releases the minimum effective dose of insulin. The sugar is shuttled into our liver, fat and muscle cells and is freed up a few hours later to exercise, heat the body, make the heart beat and thousands of other metabolic functions. You will remain lean in an insulin sensitive state.

In an insulin resistant environment It works like this: we eat sugar, our pancreas secretes insulin to signal our cells to open up and store the glucose (sugar). Because our cells are already full and resistant to insulin's effects the sugar never properly enters the cells. Our pancreas sees there is still too much sugar in the blood so it starts to secrete more and more insulin. Our fat cells finally respond to the elevated insulin levels and let the sugar in. When they stop responding the liver creates more fat cells through "de novo lipogenesis" and they too become resistant. Now you have an environment where even a small amount of sugar will cause a huge spike of insulin and brand new body fat. Finally, when your pancreas can't keep up, you'll need to take insulin shots because you have developed diabetes. This used to take decades, now it can take as little as eight weeks to move a healthy young person into prediabetes.

Here are a few other examples of how we manipulate our hormones without diet:

Testosterone Replacement Therapy (TRT): Just as prescription insulin can cause weight gain, hormone therapy is also widely used to manipulate body fat. Testosterone replacement therapy (TRT) has been shown to increase lean muscle mass while simultaneously decreasing body fat. This will happen regardless of calories, macronutrients, willpower or exercise.[5]

Thyroid: The master regulator for metabolism is your thyroid. Any dysfunction with your thyroid can lead to wild variances in metabolism and therefore your weight. Your thyroid regulates your body's metabolism by maintaining a proper balance of hormones and this is independent of any amount of calories you have eaten or used. Patients diagnosed hypothyroidism are prescribed thyroxine which helps to regulate their metabolic rate. Changing their doses will change their weight.[6]

---

[5] https://www.ncbi.nlm.nih.gov/pubmed/25105998
[6] https://www.ncbi.nlm.nih.gov/pmc/articles/PMC4044302/

Cortisol: Another prescription that can cause weight gain is prednisone. Prednisone is used as an anti-inflammatory or an immunosuppressant medication. Prednisone treats many different conditions such as allergic disorders, skin conditions, ulcerative colitis, arthritis, lupus, psoriasis, or breathing disorders. Prednisone is a synthetic hormone mimicking cortisol. Cortisol is secreted as a stress response. As we've evolved most of our stress has manifested in short bursts like running from a bear or fighting off other humans. In these fight or flight situations we are in need of a quick burst of energy. Cortisol floods our bodies and frees up glucose to be used immediately by muscle tissue. This hormone spike is designed to be short and disappear quickly.

Our stressors have changed over the last couple thousand years. For sure we still need to fight and run from things but now most of our stress is low and constant. Stress from relationships, job related stress, and freaking out about money are all constantly simmering. This raises our cortisol a small amount but keeps it elevated all day, everyday. Because of this chronic stress we have a chronic glucose drip. Because of this chronic glucose drip we have a chronic insulin response. Because of this chronic insulin response we build up a tolerance and eventually a resistance. Throw a bunch of sugar in your belly and you now have a metabolic disaster.

Prescribed a little prednisone, patients gained a little weight. Prescribed a lot of prednisone patients gain a lot of weight. Lower the dose of prednisone and patients will lose weight. Once again we observe weight gain without a calorie increase and not attributed to lack of willpower or because food is delicious.[7]

There are many other drugs that can affect your body weight regardless of how much you eat or how much you exercise but the takeaway is this: Your body weight is tightly regulated by your hormonal environment. Manipulate your hormones and you will change your body. Now that you have a bird's-eye-view of some hormones I hope you can see through the "calorie is a calorie" dogma.

Conclusion

We spend a lot of time complicating weight gain and weight loss but most of our efforts are aimed at the symptoms of weight gain not the actual cause. Blaming it on calories is essentially just blaming it on behavior but as we've seen our bodies are tightly regulated by hormones that are synced with each other and tend to influence our behavior. Almost every weight loss plan you've ever seen deals with weight gain well after the trigger point, too late into the process to

---

[7] https://www.ncbi.nlm.nih.gov/pubmed/21635675

have any lasting effect. It's like cleaning up the blood from a cut instead of closing the wound. In this program we will deal with the actual biological insult.

Section 2: How People Get Fat

In this section we will detail exactly how people get fat and the various health consequences that come along with gaining weight. More than 70% of deaths in the United States are due to chronic disease. Cardiovascular deaths, some cancer deaths, and neurodegenerative deaths have a common culprit. Fructose induced insulin resistance is at the core of all of these preventable, chronic diseases and it begins with one trigger.

A Broken Environment

If you could create a timelapse video of a healthy man gaining a hundred pounds over 30 years you would probably notice that all of his weight gain begins in the center of the body. The adipose (fat) tissue in his stomach is the first to receive excess fat and sugar from his liver. Fat will then creep out to the hypodermis (under the skin) in his limbs neck and face, looking for cells that are not already full and resistant. That is why you will never see a man with fat arms and ripped abs.

Weight gain, once triggered, will always start with the liver and the overflow will move to the closest, easiest cells to fill. Once those cells are full the next closest cells will fill up and so on. Just like a pyramid of champagne glasses at a wedding. This could be because insulin emanates from the pancreas next to the liver (where sugar and fat are released) and the closest cells are stimulated to take up glucose first and most often, this would also explain why diabetics can gain cantaloupe sized fat deposits at insulin injection sites.[8]

Now reverse the timelapse video and you will see that the fat tissue furthest from the liver and pancreas empties out first. This is also why you can't choose which body part to "tone up". If we focused on keeping our livers healthy we would not become insulin resistant or obese in the first place.

So what messes up our livers? Refined fructose.[9] The obesity epidemic directly correlates to our consumption of high fructose corn syrup along with the fructose component of regular table sugar. Our diabetes epidemic follows with a slight lag. The fructose in whole, unprocessed, unrefined fruits do not contribute to insulin resistance because they are part of what food scientist call the "food matrix", it will digest at the slower rate of the fiber it is bound to.

---

[8] http://blog.joslin.org/2015/03/ask-joslin-lumps-near-injection-sites/
[9] https://www.ncbi.nlm.nih.gov/pmc/articles/PMC4405421/

If you eat a pound of table sugar (sucrose) you are eating half a pound of glucose and half a pound of fructose. Sucrose is a 50/50 mix of glucose and fructose. The glucose half can be metabolized by every cell in your body. The fructose, on the other hand, heads straight to your liver and is converted to fat, LDL pattern B cholesterol, uric acid, and lactate. Although all sugar is at least 50% fructose, high fructose corn syrup is at least 55% fructose while agave nectar can be up to 90% fructose! Syrups are the main sweetener in beverages which make them especially fattening. Plus, there is no natural signal to prevent you from over consuming fructose. It was not present in its refined form as we evolved.

Fructose is much more readily metabolized into fat in the liver than glucose, and in the process can lead to nonalcoholic fatty liver disease.[10] NAFLD in turn leads to hepatic insulin resistance and type II diabetes. Our broken environment (insulin resistance) is directly caused by heavy and steady doses of fructose headed straight for the liver every day, all day, for years. The insulin resistant environment will overreact to stimuli including food and stress.

Foie Gras: Some people will pay a premium for this fatty duck liver. Because of this, there arose a practise of force feeding ducks sugar and refined grains specifically to fatten up their livers! All they really had to do is let those ducks follow our government's dietary guidelines and theirs livers would fatten up just like the rest of us.

Once your liver develops insulin resistance your body will follow. The liver is an important storage site for glucose, when that is compromised or full, glucose and fatty acids are shuttled to other fat storage sites like omentum (stomach fat), subcutaneous fat (under the skin), and muscle tissue in the form of glycogen. Muscle tissue is the only storage site that will not dump the glucose back into the bloodstream (because it is an engine, not a gas tank like fat tissue). The more muscle tissue you have the more sugar you can tolerate.[11]

Fatty liver always precedes insulin resistance. Insulin resistance always precedes weight gain. If your liver is insulin resistant YOU are insulin resistant. Because you are insulin resistant you will need more and more insulin in response to the same amount of glucose. This leads to more resistance. It's a vicious, fattening cycle.

---

[10] https://www.ncbi.nlm.nih.gov/pmc/articles/PMC2682989/
[11] http://jap.physiology.org/content/99/1/338

The Fat Trigger

We know that insulin causes weight gain, and that more and more insulin causes more and more weight gain, but this step doesn't come along until much later in our fat gaining process. Basically, there is a domino effect inside the liver cells that all begins with eating fructose, drinking beer, or significant breakdown of muscle tissue and ends with the cell unable to burn fat. Your body will preferentially store fat in this environment. The rest of the foods you eat that spike your insulin will only make you gain weight if this process is done first. Eating rice and potatoes will not make you obese if this process is not triggered. There are a number of very specific things that need to happen first, all inside the tiny cells in our livers. Bear with me:

1. Every second you are alive you are breaking down DNA and RNA
2. The byproducts of this degradation are converted to ATP (adenosine triphosphate)
3. You eat sugar (fructose)
4. Fructose consumes ATP breaking it down to AMP (adenosine monophosphate)[12]
5. Intracellular phosphate falls which activates AMPD (adenosine monophosphate deaminase)
6. AMPD converts to inosine monophosphate then to uric acid[13]
7. Uric acid blocks the fat metabolizing process of AMPK (adenosine monophosphate kinase)[14]
8. Uric acid stimulates fat synthesis in the hepatocyte (liver cell) and damages the mitochondria[15]
9. Insulin sensitivity drops as the cell fills up with fat and glucose
10. Your liver gets fat then you get fat
11. Your hormones command you to continue the cycle.

In nature this is a seasonal, normal process. Obesity is scheduled in many animals, they develop all the symptoms of metabolic disease. They become highly susceptible to storing energy, they become leptin resistant, their mitochondria stop fat oxidation, and their metabolic rate drops. The entire fat storing process is triggered at the end of their particular fasting cycle (e.g. end of hibernation) when they have exhausted all of their body fat and have started to break down their muscle tissue. This sets off the alarm. As muscle tissue breaks down there is significant nucleotide degradation (RNA breakdown) this causes high intracellular uric acid levels. High

---

[12] https://www.ncbi.nlm.nih.gov/books/NBK9903/
[13] https://www.sciencedaily.com/releases/2012/09/120913104121.htm
[14] https://www.ncbi.nlm.nih.gov/pmc/articles/PMC4101654/
[15] http://www.jbc.org/content/early/2012/10/03/jbc.M112.399899.full.pdf

uric acid levels stimulate aggressive foraging, raises blood pressure, activates their immune system, stimulates fat storage, and inhibits AMPK. AMPK helps you oxidize fat in your muscles and is present in very low levels in the obese and diabetic people. We want higher levels of AMPK and lower levels of AMPD for weight loss but if we eat and drink refined fructose, this cannot happen. AMPK may also contribute to tumor suppression.[16]

In the middle of a country filled up with hyper refined/ insulin spiking foods with zero satiety signals, this is a metabolic disaster. All of this is out of your control with the exception of step three. You choose to consume fructose or drink beer (with beer, it is the RNA degradation of the yeast that contributes to uric acid production) but because of the bad science and aggressive marketing blaming calories for weight gain, you had no idea that the entire obesity epidemic is essentially caused by sugar and wheat.[17]

There is a pretty good book on this mechanism called "The Fat Switch" by Richard J. Johnson MD.

Healthy Versus Broken

The difference between a person who has triggered weight gain and someone who hasn't is insulin sensitivity or resistance.The difference between insulin sensitive people (healthy) and insulin resistant people (broken) is the way their bodies react to food. If both types of people ate identical foods (calories, macros, or whatever) you would see vastly different changes in their body fat. Even though both people will have an identical increase in blood glucose the resistant person will have a significantly higher increase in insulin. Glucose is not the cause of weight gain, insulin is. All foods raise insulin to a varying degree but how your body reacts or overreacts will determine whether you get fatter on not. Overreacting to glucose by over secreting insulin leads eventually to insulin resistance, fatty liver, obesity, prediabetes and finally type II diabetes.

---

[16] https://www.ncbi.nlm.nih.gov/pmc/articles/PMC3249400/
[17] https://www.ncbi.nlm.nih.gov/pubmed/6743968/

Diabetes And Insulin Resistance

The end game of obesity is death by diabetes or diabetic complications. The reason you have to discuss diabetes when you discuss weight gain is that diabetes is the ultimate outcome if we keep getting fatter.

In type I diabetes you have what is termed "internal starvation" because the pancreas can't produce enough insulin to push the glucose into the cells. The cells never receive the energy so people start to waste away. This is why type I diabetics need exogenous (from outside the body) insulin.

According to Dr. Jason Fung (of Intensive Dietary Management in Toronto), for type II diabetes, some clinicians picture a "gummed-up" lock and key system where the key (insulin) can't fit into the keyhole (insulin receptor) so none of the glucose can get inside without major help from exogenous (outside) insulin. If they're correct we should also see the "internal starvation" present in type I diabetics, we do not. We see the opposite, the cells are overfull. The problem with this thinking is that insulin doesn't make the sugar disappear, it still has to store it somewhere. It's like sweeping the floor and putting it under the rug, you're going to have to deal with it sooner or later. The cells won't receive the glucose because there is no more room, more insulin production or injecting yourself can force it in temporarily but as soon as the insulin clears away the overflow will come spilling out.[18]

With type II diabetes, and fat gain in general, we have seen that the insulin receptor works fine (because we can sequence it) but the cell is too full to allow anymore glucose inside. When there is too much sugar and fat in the cell we start to force glucose into the least filled cells including the eyes and the kidneys. This can lead to obesity, blindness and kidney dysfunction.

Before people become diabetic they become insulin resistant. Suddenly, foods that were never a problem before are now fattening. Any foods causing a rise in insulin are now damaging. If you've never had fructose before, foods like rice, potatoes, and even milk will not cause long term weight gain. It is only after you have triggered stress in your liver and become insulin resistant that these foods become fattening. The Chinese, for example, went from a high carbohydrate diet of rice with less than 1% incidence of diabetes to an obesity and diabetes epidemic, 11.6% of the population, a few years after sugar and fructose became a dietary staple. [19] The United States comes in around 11.3% of our population diagnosed with diabetes. It is

---

[18] https://intensivedietarymanagement.com/new-paradigm-insulin-resistance-t2d/
[19] http://jamanetwork.com/journals/jama/fullarticle/1734701

interesting to note that although there are more type II diabetics in China they remain outwardly leaner than their American counterparts. There are "levels" to obesity and we have them beat, most likely due to our insatiable consumption of sugar sweetened beverages.

Sugar sweetened beverages (sweetened by HFCS) are by far the biggest contributor to insulin resistance. I personally didn't start getting fat until Starbucks opened here in Las Vegas in 1995. Daily Frappuccinos gave me a belly and my very first gout flare up at only 22 years old. I ballooned from a lean 185 lbs to over 250 lbs in just over 18 months.

The insulin hypothesis is still incomplete. It has to hold up to the same scrutiny as the energy balance theory, otherwise it's still just correlation. So why doesn't homeostasis kick in and keep the liver healthy? Because fat accumulation has been triggered at the cellular level inside the liver. Once we stop triggering it our livers will begin to heal themselves.

Your Health

I know that this isn't why you're reading this book but it is still pretty important. I need to include this section to highlight the fact that the risk for all preventable western diseases will decrease when you lose weight and become more insulin sensitive. So, not only will you lose weight on this program but the same strategies you'll use are the same strategies clinicians at the highest level are using on a daily basis to treat our greatest preventable threats: heart disease, neurological disease, diabetes, and cancer. Understanding these diseases will help you to have a better conversation with your doctor.

Sugar, diabetes and metabolic disease. The single greatest action you can take to make yourself healthier is to cut out refined sugar. Doing this alone will cause dramatic weight loss in most of us but that's not the only reason to cut it out. Sugar sweetened beverages alone can be connected to more than 180,000 deaths per year![20] Cancer, heart disease, neurological disorders, depression, diabetes, obesity, arthritis, and many more problems can all be linked back to refined sugar consumption. Starting any program that leads to reduced consumption of refined sugar will dramatically increase your health.

There are zero health consequences to totally eliminating sugar from your diet. You will never get sick and have a Doctor prescribe you cake.

For more on this I suggest you read "The Case Against Sugar" by Gary Taubes.

---

[20] http://www.cnn.com/2013/03/19/health/sugary-drinks-deaths/index.html

Cholesterol and heart disease. This is a big one. Your body needs cholesterol to create hormones, synthesize vitamin D, produce cell membranes, create enzymes used in digestion, and much more. Every cell in your body is capable of creating it. Sadly, there are a lot of clinicians that have a very low understanding of it except to prescribe cholesterol lowering drugs like statins. Dietary cholesterol does almost nothing to your body's serum cholesterol. Eating foods high in cholesterol does not change your numbers.

Knowing someone's total cholesterol number gives you zero actionable information. So, when your Doctor tells you your cholesterol is high, it's time to discuss particle size because he is likely play "risk factor bingo" versus actually checking for damage.

We know that HDL is "good" cholesterol but we also think we know that LDL is "bad" cholesterol. The problem is most clinicians don't take particle size into account before prescribing interventions.

LDL particles can be broken down into groups A and B (apolipoprotein b). The particularly harmful particle B are very small and dense and can be damaged leading to a build up in the arteries (plaque). These are created in large part by fructose (syrups not whole fruits), the problem with these smaller particles is that they are not cleared out by the liver so they tend to stick around in the body longer, because their receptor sites are partially obscured they are not easily endocytosed, giving them more of a chance to morph and cause plaques.[21]

LDL pattern A are large and buoyant and help to clear some of these smaller, damaged particles out of your system plus, a ton of other positive things in your body, including helping your body repair itself during autophagy while you are fasting.

So, if you only have a high total LDL count, and all other markers are perfect, should you take any interventions? Should you be prescribed a potentially harmful drug?

If you're concerned about heart disease you can ask your Doctor to order a test that measures particle size. There are a variety of test your doctor can order for you (depending on which lab accepts your insurance), Quest Diagnostics has a great one called the "Ion Mobility" test.

Instead of total cholesterol, here are some more reliable ways to measure heart disease risk:

1. HDL to triglycerides ratio. This should be 1:1. If your HDL is 50 than your triglycerides should be around 50. People at risk may have a 1:3 ratio or higher (HDL 50 and triglycerides 150).[22]

---

[21] http://ajcn.nutrition.org/content/86/4/1174.full
[22] https://www.ncbi.nlm.nih.gov/pmc/articles/PMC2664115/

2. CRP. C-reactive proteins are a marker of inflammation in the body. Inflammation is an essential part of your body's defense systems, if you get hurt or sick this number is high. If you're not hurt or sick it should be low. If your CRP's are chronically elevated you may have a problem.[23]

3. High Pattern B LDL particle count. These little particles can be the source of inflamed arteries leading to Atherosclerosis.[24]

If all of these markers are good then it is likely that high total cholesterol is not a concern.

Low cholesterol (below 160) has also been linked to increased all cause mortality (death by every other disease including cancer).[25]

For more on this I suggest you read "The Great Cholesterol Myth" by Jonny Bowden and Stephen Sinatra

Alternatively, there is a relatively inexpensive test that has been shown to predict heart disease far more accurately than anything most clinicians will prescribe you. The test is known as the Coronary Artery Calcium (CAC) test. It is performed by taking an ultrafast Computerized Tomogram (CT) scan of your chest. The more calcium, the greater the amount of damaging cholesterol buildup in your heart arteries, which is what causes heart attacks. The test takes about 30 minutes. Most health insurance plans don't pay for coronary calcium scanning. The cost can range from about $100 to $400. Calcium buildup in the arteries has been linked to hyperinsulinemia. The more insulin resistant you are, the more likely you are to have a high calcium score, diabetes, and heart disease.[26]

Cancer: There are many correlative studies between meat eating and cancer but in every single study, subjects had at least one other factor involved, for example: high sugar diets, smoking, exposure to carcinogens, heavy alcohol consumption, heavy sun overexposure (sunburns), or a sedentary lifestyle. Cancer needs two things to thrive: an initiation event and an environment to thrive and grow. A high sugar and/ or a high meat diet can create an environment for cancer to grow. Meat consumption, by itself, is not an initiator and does not appear to cause cancer but it may help it grow (through IGF-1) once it is initiated.[27][28][29]

There is an increasing number of researchers subscribing to the metabolic theory of cancer initiation. Otherwise known as the Warburg Effect, this theory postulates that cancer is caused by the fermentation of sugar in the mitochondria while oxygen is present. Both fasting and a

---

[23] http://circ.ahajournals.org/content/107/3/363

[24] https://www.ncbi.nlm.nih.gov/pubmed/15296705

[25] http://www.medscape.com/viewarticle/786515

[26] https://www.nhlbi.nih.gov/health/health-topics/topics/cscan

[27] https://www.ncbi.nlm.nih.gov/pmc/articles/PMC2527479/

[28] https://bmcmedicine.biomedcentral.com/articles/10.1186/1741-7015-11-63

[29] http://ajcn.nutrition.org/content/89/5/1620S.long

ketogenic diet have had tremendous effects on not only lowering risk factors but also slowing tumor growth, and helping relieve some of the adverse effects of chemotherapy.[30]

For more on this I suggest reading "Tripping Over The Truth" by Travis Christofferson.

Better health As A Side Effect

The same steps you would take to lose weight on this program are the same steps clinicians are using to combat and help prevent all chronic western diseases. Fasting and the ketogenic diet are being used to treat cancer and side effects of chemotherapy, seizures, alzheimer's and other neurological disorders, type II diabetes, and high blood pressure. There is even a small group of clinicians using these therapies for dogs! Check out ketopetsanctuary.com for more information. If you are a human and you are suffering from diabetes there is also a group designed to help you in your fight, check out virtahealth.com for more information.

---

[30] https://www.ncbi.nlm.nih.gov/pmc/articles/PMC2849637/

How People Get Fat

Let's go step-by-step and re-enact exactly what it takes to go from being lean and healthy to suffering from obesity and diabetes.

The starting point varies for everyone for a few reasons. For instance, if your Mother is overweight there will be physical biological differences from a baby born to lean parents. Also, even if your Mother was lean, what she ate when you were being developed will determine how you react or overreact to certain foods. A woman with gestational diabetes can give birth to a child with fetal macrosomia, a greater amount of insulin secreting beta cells in its pancreas, and insulin resistance in its liver. This is likely why babies are getting fatter and fatter every year.

For this example, we are not going to start with a fat baby. We will assume our baby is born with an average weight to average weight parents.

Babies

As parents start to introduce foods to a baby one-at-a-time, they notice that most babies will respond positively to sweeter foods. When you have a tired or busy mom she will default to what her baby likes rather than having a teaching moment when she is in a hurry. When this behavior continues into the toddler years you see three-year-olds drinking apple juice, Capri Sun, and eating handfuls of Cheerios or a packaged fruit mush (mostly just liquid fructose).

Toddlers

Although some kids will start gaining fat far over normal levels even as they start kindergarten there are kids at this age that will remain lean for now. This is likely due to certain genetic polymorphisms to insulin sensitivity and a rush of human growth hormone. It is at this point that highly refined breakfast cereals enter the picture, along with sodas, sandwiches and constant snacks made from refined sugar, wheat and corn. Seriously, go to any baby aisle in any store, it's all highly refined, super palatable crap. Now they have an internal environment primed for fat storage but for most, their growth hormones will keep them relatively lean.

Pre Teens

It is at this point that over 200,000 kids will be diagnosed with juvenile type II diabetes, a term that would have made zero sense thirty-years-ago. Every single food marketed to children this age is packed with refined sugar, wheat, or corn syrup. This is also the age parents will notice that their kid is a little, or even a lot, fatter than the other kids. It is important to note that even with a high sugar diet and their obesity being triggered some kids will remain average size while they are maturing. By the way, kids are mean and their insults could help shape other kid's self esteem.

Another new disease that kids this age need to deal with is non-alcoholic fatty liver disease (NAFLD). We know that the liver is the first organ affected by metabolic disease and we know that fructose directly contributes to this condition. If steps are not taken at this point to reverse this condition (or it remains undiagnosed) that kid runs the risk of developing a variety of western diseases, both physical and neurological. Parents and pediatricians should take an honest assessment of a child's body composition and determine if they are carrying true baby fat and will lean out in their teens or if there is liver dysfunction worsening with every teaspoon of sugar they eat. If NAFLD is an option a pediatrician will check the kid's fasting glucose and insulin response followed by an invasive liver biopsy. Kids should not have to go through this and if they avoid fructose, they won't need to.

Teenagers

As puberty hits, most kids (not all) see a drop in body fat and tend to lean out as sex hormones take control and begin to regulate metabolism. These eight years or so are the glory days for their body composition as they tend to be able to eat whatever they want to with seemingly zero consequences. What they are actually doing, if they haven't done it as a toddler, is priming their bodies for a metabolic storm that is about to hit. At this age almost everything kids do involves having a sugary drink in their hand. Gatorade, energy drinks, big gulps, and now Frappuccinos are all high fructose delivery systems. The fructose in these drinks go straight to the liver, constantly triggering fat storage while the glucose from these drinks and other snacks causes a near constant insulin release.

What has likely happened at this point is that they have triggered fat storage over and over with a high consumption of fructose, from here the only mechanism keeping some of them from obesity is the super high prevalence of growth hormones and testosterone. Fat storage for some people becomes secondary to actually maturing. For kids that are already obese at this point you will see significantly lower levels testosterone (an effect of sugar consumption).

Studies have shown that as little as 75 grams of sugar (a small donut and a soda) can decrease testosterone by as much as 25% over the next few hours. So, 75 grams of sugar every three or four hours for years is going to have a dramatic effect of their body composition regardless of them being in the golden age of metabolism.

Young Adults

Let's say they made it through high school with their waistlines intact. At the college age they will experience a drop in the hormones that were holding back their weight gain because they have reached a genetically predisposed height and weight. This is where we see the "freshman fifteen" phenomenon, a period when college freshman gain fifteen pounds or more in a semester. You see, their fat storage is still triggered but now the opposing hormones are fading and they will continue to fade year after year. Their diet hasn't changed, it's still highly refined wheat and sugar (and now alcohol), but now they have no protection against its effects and their hijacked livers are signalling that winter and famine is coming the same way it always has for hundreds-of-thousands-of-years. These are the years of fast, cheap food, energy drinks, and sugary coffee.

30 Somethings

Sometimes it's an unflattering reflection, a comment from a friend or moving up in clothes sizes that open their eyes to the weight gain. This is likely the point when most people have a heart to heart with themselves and begin to take more responsibility for their bodies. With absolutely zero research they plunge into a diet and exercise program. The program they choose seems intuitive, plus it has been rammed down their throats for decades (even as obesity has steadily increased in lockstep with these guidelines). They opt for the Biggest Loser style "eat less, move more" strategy. So they start their diet and cut back on almost all of the most obvious offenders (ice cream, regular soda) and instead choose low fat foods and diet drinks.

Because of where they are starting their regimen, they will see immediate success. Having started a cardio routine and avoiding cupcakes like the plague they see ten pounds melt away almost effortlessly. The next ten pounds proves to be a little more stubborn though so they cut way back on their calories and jog a little further everyday.

They lose a little less weight every time but the less results they see the harder they work. It's at this point that most of them give up and start over next January, every year. Because they did not address the real cause of their weight gain, all of the weight they lost comes back quickly. The worst part is their resting metabolic rate (RMR) has slowed with this strategy and isn't bouncing back as fast. Just like the Biggest Loser contestants.

They intuitively stick with the diet soda and low fat foods (as we know, low fat means high sugar) but they are eating more of them than they used to. They are stuck in the lower calorie mindset even though it has failed them (and everyone else) for decades.

40 to 50 year olds

The weight gain continues to soar. This is where life gets kind of scary. A lifetime of high fructose and refined food consumption has fattened them up, and they have learned to accept that, but now they have a frightening visit with their doctor.

In a six to ten minute visit he reviews their blood work with them. He tells them unfamiliar numbers and abbreviations but the only thing most of them understand is their cholesterol is too high (even though they are not sure what cholesterol is). He goes on to explain that they have high blood pressure, high triglycerides and a prediabetic HBA1C level. On their way out he mentions they may have a fatty liver and reminds them that they'll discuss it at the next visit.

They finally leave their doctor's office with a prescription for statin drugs, the advice to eat less and exercise more, and an appointment for a follow up visit. At the follow up visit, a few months later, if there is no improvement with the high blood pressure and HBA1C, they will likely be prescribed pills for those too. Some clinicians will also give you a "heart healthy" low fat diet plan printed out from the American Heart Association's website or the DASH (dietary approach to stop hypertension) plan.

This is the age where most diabetes diagnoses occur. Along with this diagnosis comes a myriad of prescriptions including insulin. The more insulin prescribed, the fatter they get.

People over 50

For this example, this is as far as we are going to go. The sixties is just other people taking care of you and there probably won't be many seventies (if any). This is going to be a decade of pills, injections, blood work and doctor visits.

For most people in the U.S. all of the symptoms they are being medicated for (and all of the side effects of those potentially harmful prescriptions) can be linked to hyperinsulinemia, which itself is a symptom of triggered weight gain.

Despite the medications, they are likely to suffer a cardiac event which will lead to greater lifestyle restrictions. There is also the probability that their diabetes will worsen over time with continued insulin injections and may lead to blindness or the loss of one or both legs.

This is misery. I've seen it. I've lived it. I wouldn't wish it on anyone but each of us know dozens of people who live this everyday.

Conclusion

Now imagine that the person in this example isn't some stranger. It isn't even you. Instead, imagine it is your son or daughter. What would you give to go back to your three-year-old and take back the sippy cup full of apple juice? As a parent, you provide the trigger for fat storage and you are 100% in control of whether or not they are raised in an environment for obesity to thrive. Fix it.

The good news is, no matter where you may be in this example, you can still turn the fat signal off, shed all those extra pounds, and live the rest of your life lean and healthy.

Section 3: Weight Loss For People In A Hurry

In this section we will go step-by-step and use the knowledge we just gained to drop weight as fast as humanly possible, change our internal environment so that it will be extremely difficult to gain any weight back, and lay the foundation for a longer healthier life.

The Fat Burning Trigger

We now know that fat storage can be triggered (we can observe it happen in a cell) and that this is a necessary evolutionary biological process, but what about triggering fat loss? Is there an evolutionary biological mechanism for that? Fat storage is energy storage. When in our evolution have we had to access these stores? More specifically, is there a mechanism we can observe that causes the purging of our stored body fat?

If you want to take glucose out of a fat cell and put it into circulation where it can be used by your muscles or other resting biological functions (like thinking, breathing, or raising your body temperature), you are going to want your liver to release a healthy dose of glucagon.

How do you release glucagon? Stop eating. Glucagon is the opposite of insulin and their balance is necessary to regulate blood glucose levels. The downside is that if your metabolism is slowed down, that glucose stays in circulation and eventually get shuttled back into the fats cells.[31] If our metabolism is turned up that circulating glucose can get shuttled into cells that will actually use it like your organs, muscles, and brain. Our next step is obviously to increase our metabolism (RMR) or at least to prevent it from crashing.

The single greatest action you can take to burn fat and keep it off is to raise your resting metabolic rate (RMR). How can we raise our RMR? We can build muscle but that takes a lot of time and this is Weight Loss For People In A Hurry. So, without waiting to pack on some lean muscle is there a faster way? Indeed, it's called adrenaline.

If you want your RMR to jump through the roof try being chased by a tiger. The resulting cascade of adrenaline will rip through your fat stores and make you feel like you put rocket fuel in your espresso and injected it into your veins.[32] This is an all or nothing scenario to stay alive

---

[31] https://www.ncbi.nlm.nih.gov/pmc/articles/PMC3432929/
[32] https://www.ncbi.nlm.nih.gov/pubmed/6380304

followed by a huge hangover. We can opt for a slightly more subtle rise in adrenaline by just not eating.

When you stop eating, adrenalin levels are increased so that we have plenty of energy to go get more food. For example, forty-eight hours of fasting produces a 3.6% increase in metabolic rate.[33] In response to a four day fast, RMR increased up to 14%. Rather than slowing the metabolism down, instead the body speeds it up.

In short, burning fat is our default mode and our fat burning switch is just to stop eating. If we could just get out of our own way, our body fat will melt off very quickly, but without the right strategies, this can seem almost impossible.

Moving Forward

We need to turn off the fat trigger and focus on restoring our livers to their former glory. Our livers are directly and indirectly responsible for more than five hundred individual functions in our bodies. When our livers are packed full of sugar and fatty acids this affects our daily lives. Our sleep, our skin, our mood, and our longevity all depend on our livers to function normally. So, after years of attacking them with fructose, we need to let them heal.

The good news is our livers are surprisingly resilient and can regenerate themselves. If you were to cut off a huge piece of your liver and throw it away, this organ would re-grow very quickly without missing a beat in its daily functions.[34] The bad news is cutting your liver up is not an option so, you're going to have to do it the hard way. The hard way consists of changing your diet and habits in an attempt to empty your liver of fat and sugar.

We also need to heal our mitochondria. Some of the mitochondria in obese people have completely given up on metabolizing fat and instead can only churn out energy from burning glucose.[35] It's easy enough to starve these particular cells of sugar and let apoptosis handle the rest.

Apoptosis is programmed cell death. There are checkpoints in a cell's natural cycle that will cause the cell to die off when it is damaged or useless. When this function is overridden and the

---

[33] https://intensivedietarymanagement.com/fasting-physiology-part-ii/
[34] https://www.ncbi.nlm.nih.gov/pmc/articles/PMC2701258/
[35] https://www.ncbi.nlm.nih.gov/pmc/articles/PMC4765362/

damaged cell lives on past these checkpoints, this is the beginning of tumor growth and can eventually lead to (or be caused by) cancer.[36]

The first step toward insulin sensitivity is to stop the behaviors that made us resistant in the first place. Adjust the foods we eat as outlined in the "what to eat" section of this manual. Once we have our habits tweaked, and we have stopped causing the damage, then we can begin repairing our livers.

By far the best way to repair our bodies is to get out of the way and let our bodies heal themselves. The body's natural repair mechanism is a process called autophagy and it occurs while we are fasted. The effectiveness of autophagy increases with time spent in a fasted state.[37] These same processes stop when we are in a fed state.

Fasting

Fasting is voluntarily going without food for a set amount of time.

The single greatest dietary intervention to prevent disease and reduce body fat is fasting. Fasting differs from caloric restriction in a few key ways. Fasting triggers numerous hormonal adaptations that do NOT happen with simple caloric reduction. When you fast, insulin drops precipitously, helping prevent insulin resistance. Noradrenalin rises, keeping metabolism high. Growth hormone rises to maintain lean mass, and glucagon levels rise specifically targeting the sugar/ fat storage in your liver.

Glucagon is a glucose retrieving hormone. Glucagon and insulin are like day and night. If insulin rises, glucagon subsides. If insulin levels lower, glucagon comes out. This process is an important balancing act for the liver to keep your blood sugar at healthy levels. When insulin is done storing everything, glucagon goes to the liver to free up some fatty acids and glucose to use as energy. This process is key to reversing hepatic (liver related) insulin resistance. If we don't let this happen often enough our livers will just keep getting fatter and sicker.

This is really quite interesting. Fasting, but not low calorie diets results in numerous hormonal adaptations that all appear to be highly beneficial on many levels. In essence, fasting transitions the body from burning sugar to burning fat. Resting metabolism is NOT decreased but instead increased. We are, effectively, feeding our bodies through our own fat. We are 'eating' our own

---

[36] https://www.ncbi.nlm.nih.gov/pmc/articles/PMC4925817/
[37] https://www.ncbi.nlm.nih.gov/pmc/articles/PMC3106288/

fat. This makes total sense. Fat, in essence is stored food. In fact, studies show that the epinephrine (adrenalin) induced fat burning does not depend upon lowering blood sugar.

How does adrenaline work in the body?
Key actions of adrenaline include increasing the heart rate, increasing blood pressure, expanding the air passages of the lungs, enlarging the pupil in the eye, redistributing blood to the muscles and altering the body's metabolism, so as to maximise blood glucose levels (primarily for the brain)"

With a calorie restricted diet you will lower the amount of glucose in a cell but you constantly replenish this when you eat your low-calorie diet. Insulin may be lower than usual but still present. You cannot metabolize fat with insulin present. When you are in a constantly fed state you will rarely dip into your fat stores for energy, your glucagon levels never rise, your basal-metabolic rate drops, and every function in your body slows to a crawl with your new lower resting metabolic rate.

In a fasted state you will burn through your glucose stores very quickly and in less than twenty-four hours you will be converting your stored body fat to energy. This happens to most of us, to a lesser extent, everyday. Unless you are already diabetic or if you haven't slept long enough (more on that later) you are burning body fat when you wake up every morning. You will continue to burn a little more body fat all day, until you eat.

Prolonged fasting benefits: dramatic boost in autophagy and apoptosis followed by a massive boost in stem cell production. Not to mention fasting induced apoptosis can prevent damaged cells from becoming cancer cells.[38]

One of the biggest concerns about fasting is muscle loss. I always hear that you're going to lose all of your muscle if you fast. This is just wrong and ridiculous. You will not burn protein from muscle tissue while you fast until you run out of fat stores (as is the case with physique competitors). There are studies showing a slight increase in muscle mass after a four to five day fast. This is due to an increase in growth hormone. If our muscle tissue deteriorated while fasting we would not be around as a species right now. Why would we store energy as fat if we were just going to use protein from our muscles? It's a ridiculous argument with zero scientific backing. You will, however, lose some water causing your muscles to look "flatter". This look is immediately reversed when you refeed or break your fast.[39]

[38] http://www.sciencemag.org/news/2017/02/five-day-fasting-diet-could-fight-disease-slow-aging
[39] https://www.ncbi.nlm.nih.gov/pubmed/11147801

While fasted, your brain can very quickly switch over to using body fat for fuel in the form of ketones, this strategy is being used to treat a myriad of neurological disorders by clinicians across the globe.[40][41] There is a subculture of people that use this strategy as a lifestyle. They use what is termed a ketogenic diet to stay in ketosis. Not to be confused with diabetic ketoacidosis, which can be fatal.

Ketosis is being successfully used to treat everything from neurological disorders like seizures and alzheimer's to cancer growth and metabolic diseases like diabetes and obesity. You will enter ketosis on this program. During ketosis uric acid goes way down, AMPK (adenosine monophosphate kinase) goes up. There are also people treating dogs for cancer and seizure disorders at Ketopetsanctuary.com using a ketogenic diet.

The problem with fasting is that if you tell anyone you're fasting they'll give you a million reasons why they think it's a bad idea. Those same people will happily order a pizza and drink some beer with you. If you happened to catch a cold, get in an argument or have a bad night's sleep, your friends will blame it on fasting. The best thing you can do is just do your thing and not announce your fast to the people that might try to sabotage you.

Fasting is vilified for a few reasons the most common being; there is no way to profit from it (you can't sell fasting), this is the reason funding for studies is hard to come by. Companies that produce products are not interested in funding studies that can't possible lead to producing profitable products. Also, there are IRB's (institutional review boards) and other ethics committees that will never approve a study that they believe is unethical and/ or unprofitable.

Another concern is that you'll take it too far and become anorexic. Anorexia is a neurological issue not a dietary side effect. The mental disorder will or will not exist despite how you choose to eat, fasting and anorexia are not related.

Without a doubt, you will lose weight when you fast, you will preserve muscle, you will lower your body's "fat thermostat" (RMR), and your body will start to repair itself through a process called autophagy. At the end of the day YOU MUST BE IN A FASTED STATE TO REPAIR DAMAGE, which is why most repairs occur while you are sleeping. That is the only time most people are in a fasted state.

If you're thinking about giving prolonged fasting a shot, run it by a medical doctor. Women who are pregnant or nursing should not fast. Children should not fast. People that are generally undernourished should not fast.

---

[40] https://www.ncbi.nlm.nih.gov/pmc/articles/PMC3946160/
[41] https://www.ncbi.nlm.nih.gov/pmc/articles/PMC3321471/

Autophagy

Autophagy is damage repair at the cellular level that only occurs while fasted.

The 2016 recipient of the Nobel prize for physiology or medicine is Yoshinori Ohsumi. His discovery: Ohsumi studied the function of the proteins encoded by key autophagy genes. He delineated how stress signals initiate autophagy and the mechanism by which proteins and protein complexes promote distinct stages of autophagosome formation.

Autophagy is a cellular clean up mechanism. Inside each cell there are degraded products left over from stress. Autophagosomes move the debri into the lysosomes where they can be broken down for energy or stripped of parts to be reused.[42] It is essentially an anti-aging process. Disrupted autophagy has been linked to Parkinson's disease, type II diabetes and other disorders that appear in the elderly.[43] Mutations in autophagy genes can cause genetic disease. Disturbances in the autophagic machinery have also been linked to cancer. Intense research is now ongoing to develop drugs that can target autophagy in various diseases.

The level of autophagy activity can be measured by simply counting the number of autophagosomes (the cellular organelles that degrade dysfunctional proteins) present in the cell, as these will increase in number when autophagy is stimulated. The study looking at liver cells found that the number of autophagosomes increased 300% after 24 hours of fasting, and a further 30% after 48 hours of fasting (remember we are trying to repair our livers). Studies looking at autophagosomes in brain cells had similar findings. Autophagy repairs your liver, brain, and everything else in your body. Damaged mitochondria are preferentially selected by autophagy, which is crucial to fixing our metabolism.[44][45]

In short, if you leave your body alone, it will start to fix itself. Fasting induced autophagy doesn't just target cellular junk but also unnecessary cells. Your organs can shrink when you are fasting. Cells won't just temporarily empty out (like with a calorie restricted diet) they actually die (apoptosis) and get recycled (autophagy). When you stop fasting and refeed, you will have a new "set point" for body fat. So now, your body's homeostatic mechanism will fight like hell to keep your body at your new weight instead of forcing you to gain the weight back. That is the key

---

[42] http://stke.sciencemag.org/content/4/178/ec175
[43] https://translationalneurodegeneration.biomedcentral.com/articles/10.1186/s40035-016-0065-1
[44] https://www.ncbi.nlm.nih.gov/pmc/articles/PMC3439916/
[45] https://www.ncbi.nlm.nih.gov/pmc/articles/PMC3748187/

difference between weight loss on a calorie restricted diet and weight loss from a fasting protocol.[46]

Satiety

What can you eat that will make you not want to eat for awhile? How much milk can you drink before your body screams at you to stop? How many apples can you grind through? Contrast that with accidentally polishing off a full bag of cheetos or a pint of ice cream while watching a twenty-two minute sitcom, and you'll understand the role satiety plays in weight gain and weight loss.

All whole, unprocessed, or minimally processed foods will signal you to stop eating them. Highly refined foods have these mechanisms removed for profit. If you want to sell a lot of food you just need to strip it of fiber and fill it up with sugar. If you've ever eaten a sleeve of Oreos then you know exactly what I mean.

Manipulating your satiety hormones is a crucial first step to weight loss. Unfortunately, this step is almost always ignored by most weight loss plans. Being hungry versus not being hungry seems to be the war people wage with themselves and why some weight loss programs can cause emotional meltdowns, crying and yelling. When it comes to fat loss, the battle in between meals is where the war is won or lost. Your meals have to make you not want to eat for awhile. Your food should prepare you to function without food. This is all important when it comes to fasting.

We all know about sugar causing spikes and crashes but we rarely think about which foods actually keep us full. Usually, we think of satiety depending on an amount of food we eat, not an effect of a certain food. If you want to increase the time between bouts of hunger than you would definitely choose to eat a steak and green beans over a bowl of pasta. This leads us to fasting, or more specifically, which foods to eat before you don't eat for awhile. The hormones we need to keep us from being hungry are the results of what we have eaten in the past few days.

There are a wide variety of satiety hormones, here are the top two:
Cholecystokinin (CKK): as a peptide hormone, CCK mediates satiety by acting on the CCK receptors distributed widely throughout the central nervous system. The mechanism for hunger suppression is thought to be a decrease in the rate of gastric emptying. When you eat fats CKK will slow digestion which can signal the brain, via the vagus nerve, to stop eating.[47]

---

[46] https://www.sciencedaily.com/releases/2016/05/160509085347.htm
[47] https://www.ncbi.nlm.nih.gov/pubmed/16246215

Leptin: Leptin is secreted by your body's fat cells in response to insulin. It sends a message to your brain letting you know that you have enough fat stored so you won't need to eat right now. The message is simply to stop storing and start using energy. Leptin and insulin both signal our brains via the vagus nerve but insulin will always receive preferential treatment, probably because we will die without proper insulin signalling. If you are insulin resistant there is a good chance you are also leptin resistant. Leptin resistance is one of the reasons most of us plateau with weight loss on traditional diets.[48][49]

Now that we know that we have to aggressively stimulate our satiety hormones, the question becomes: what foods should we use to do it?

[48] https://www.ncbi.nlm.nih.gov/pubmed/17212793
[49] http://legacy.lakeforest.edu/images/userImages/eukaryon/Page_7943/20_R_Pospiech.pdf

How To Eat

Before you start this program I want you to really feel what it's like to not want to eat. Pick an unprocessed food (apples, broccoli, cheese, steak) and eat as much of it as you can. Once you get to the point that taking another bite feels like it would take a tremendous amount of willpower, then you know you have successfully activated your satiety hormones. Do you feel how hard it is to eat more? Digging deep and exhausting your willpower can get you through a couple more bites but you will eventually have to give in, your hormones take over the decision making at this point.

This is exactly how hard it is to not eat sugar and wheat when you are on a high sugar diet. You can dig deep again and hold out for a little while but eventually you're going to eat some cookies. Fighting against your hormones will always end in defeat. We can however, plan against them days or even minutes before the battle begins by getting full on the right foods.

When To Eat

When we eat is at least as important as what we eat. There have been studies that have changed only the timing of meals with the exact same foods that have resulted in dramatically different results in weight loss. Balancing fasting with feeding seems to be the way we have evolved.

We know that we are going to have to fast at some point but we can't jump right into it without severe side effects. For this program it is important to learn how to manipulate our satiety hormones before we even think about abstaining from food. The time between each meal is the only time you can possibly dip into your body fat stores. The foods that we eat should help us spread each meal out to maximize fat metabolism.

Extended fasting can be as little as 24 hours to a record 382 days, this guy reported a sense of well being the entire time.[50] He was medically supervised and his doctors reported no ill effects. He started the fast at 454 lbs and ended at about 185 lbs. One of the most notable benefits was that he did not end up with a bunch of excess skin typically seen with weight loss from low calorie diets. This is likely due to autophagy and the breakdown and recycling of unnecessary cells. With each day fasted a whole different level of cellular clean up can occur.

---

[50] https://www.ncbi.nlm.nih.gov/pmc/articles/PMC2495396/pdf/postmedj00315-0056.pdf

Aside from extended fasting there are other strategies that may fit your life better. This is where intermittent fasting (or time restricted feeding) comes in. For this program we will focus on the 16:8 style. Choose an eight hour window and don't eat outside of that. For example if you choose to eat between the hours of 12PM to 8PM you will fast until 12PM the next day. sixteen hours fasted and eight hours fed. Keep in mind the hormonal benefits and autophagy compound with each consecutive hour of fasting.

For optimal weight loss the earlier in the day you start your eating window the faster you will lose weight. Some of the same genes that regulate our metabolism are linked to our circadian rhythm (sleep wake cycle). For optimal compliance though, I've found that putting off eating is ten times easier than actually stopping eating for the day. Choose whatever time fits your lifestyle.

What To Eat

There are two extremes you can aim for when it comes to your diet but most of us will probably land right in the middle.

For a few of us (not recommended for beginners). The first extreme is to be as diligent as possible when it comes to micronutrients (Vitamins and minerals) to prevent any nutrient deficiencies. You'll have to be super strict about where your food comes from and may even have to take supplements depending on what time of year it is and where you live. Once you start going down this rabbit hole you'll see that most of the people that are this detailed about their intake usually have a "go to" smoothie recipe that they power down every day.

Here's an example from one of my favorite scientists, Dr. Rhonda Patrick's daily smoothie:
Serving Size is ~64 fluid ounces (1.9 liters)
Ingredients (All Organic):
8 large kale leaves (I use an entire bunch of curly kale). 4-6 rainbow chard leaves with stems
3 cups (~710 ml) of baby spinach (a large handful)
2 medium to large carrots
1 tomato
1 large avocado
1 banana
1 apple
1 cup (~710ml) of blueberries (fresh or frozen)
1 tall shot glass of flaxseed (optional)

3 cups (~710 ml) of unsweetened flax milk

She goes on to explain each ingredient in detail and its effects on the body on her website. Foundmyfitness.com. This with properly sourced fish, a variety of vegetables, and laser focus on supplementation based on blood test results can dramatically increase your health and lifespan. This micronutrient strategy might be in some of our futures but for right now we need to just lose weight.

For the rest of us. At the other end of the spectrum we can be more cavalier with our meals. We just need to get some vegetable fiber, some fat, and some meat then eat enough so that we don't want to eat for awhile. When dealing with the real world, pre-packaged frozen vegetables and meat along with fast food will make up a significant part of our diets.

Vegetables and Fruit. It would be nice to have a garden. You could just walk out, grab some fresh leafy greens, clean them off in the sink with a special produce brush and some vegetable wash that you can get from Whole foods. It would be nice….not necessary.

If you're like the rest of us you could just pop a frozen Green Giant Broccoli Steamer in the microwave for five minutes. They will both have the same effect on your insulin and as for nutrition, studies have shown over and over that they are essentially the same.[51] There are multiple references in published medical journals you can read or if you just want the basics, the New York Times published several articles about this.[52][53] Frozen vegetables are as nutritious as fresh vegetables.[54] So, don't let anyone be a dick about it. Eat either one.

Frozen vegetables are super cheap and really quick with almost no clean up. There is no excuse to not get your veggies in. Just don't get the products mixed with pasta or rice.

For smoothies, don't juice, just blend if you want. You need the fiber, especially with fruit. Juicing fruits is just as bad for fat loss as drinking a Dr. Pepper, it just becomes vitamin syrup. Not only do you need the micronutrients (vitamins) in vegetables to survive but you also need the fiber. The fiber in vegetables is essential for satiety and keeping the bacteria that reside in your colon healthy. Why do you care about these little bugs? Simple, they can manipulate your hormones better than you can.

---

[51] https://www.ncbi.nlm.nih.gov/pubmed/?term=27211670
[52] https://well.blogs.nytimes.com/2016/11/18/are-frozen-fruits-and-vegetables-as-nutritious-as-fresh/
[53] https://well.blogs.nytimes.com/ask/well/questions/eat-well
[54] https://www.ncbi.nlm.nih.gov/pubmed/25526594

For the sake of brevity, we will divide your gut bacteria into two categories: Harmful and beneficial. The harmful bacteria feed on glucose and other sugars that you eat.[55] When they over grow the beneficial bacteria you will crave more and more refined sugar and wheat. The beneficial bacteria help fight off infections, improve your mood, energy, and insulin sensitivity. They feed on what we call prebiotic fiber from vegetables, seeds and nuts.

Vegetable and fruit fiber can slow gastric emptying and increase satiety while feeding these beneficial bacteria.[56][57] It has also been shown to attenuate the insulin response you would normally get from food. This is why eating apples won't make you fat, and why you can't eat more than a couple of them.[58]

Replacing fiberless foods with vegetable fiber is a must for any weight loss program. You have to do this. Just pick the foods you like and eat them over and over, variety can be the enemy of consistency.

Eat: Broccoli, Kale, Spinach, Brussels sprouts, Chard, Green beans, Peas, Cauliflower, Corn, Carrots, Lettuce, Pickles, Tomatoes, Olives, Sweet potatoes, Broccolini, Alfalfa sprouts, Onions, Bell peppers, Jalapenos, Zucchini, Squash, Mushrooms, Apples, Bananas, All berries, Melon, Avocado, Oranges, Watermelon, Grapes, Raisins, Pears, Plums, Peaches, etc.

Basic green smoothie: kale or spinach or both, and almond or coconut milk. Add any whole fruits or berries for taste. You can get as fancy as you want with these, just don't add sugar.

Meat. I like more expensive meat (title of your sex tape). It's probably due to my time in the restaurant industry. Don't let that stop you, when it comes to weight loss eat whatever meat you want. Lunch meat is a great snack, beef jerky is amazingly convenient, or just get a "protein style" (no bun) burger from any drive through. Don't get fries.

Hamburgers, chicken, turkey, pork, fish, sausages, bacon or straight up eating a steak are all fine. If you're on a budget get frozen meats. The hardest thing about the protein you choose is figuring out the sugar content of any sauces you want to use. Most BBQ sauces and even ketchups are really high in sugar, don't eat those.

Grass fed beef has a more favorable fat profile and can provide health benefits over time. The problem is that is costs way more. If you can get grass-fed beef and wild caught fish you

---

[55] https://www.ncbi.nlm.nih.gov/pmc/articles/PMC3448089/
[56] http://gut.bmj.com/content/gutjnl/36/6/825.full.pdf
[57] https://www.ncbi.nlm.nih.gov/pmc/articles/PMC3705355/
[58] https://www.ncbi.nlm.nih.gov/pubmed/71495

probably should but for weight loss it just doesn't matter that much. Fatty meats are the best due to the increased satiety effect of saturated fat and as a benefit, all fats tend to help lower the insulin rise you will get from meat.[59]

Meat consumption increases IGF-1 (insulin-like growth factor 1). IGF-1 will help you preserve muscle while decreasing your fat tissue. Meat consumption also signals the brain to stop eating after ingesting a small amount, you can override this signal by eating sugar. Which is why a lot of packaged meats contain hidden and not so hidden sugars.[60]

Eat: Ham, Steak, Ground beef, Sausage, Bacon, Chicken, Pork, Lamb, Turkey, Duck, Hot dogs, Roast beef, Lunch meat, Beef jerky, Tuna, Salmon, Cod, Liver, Salami, Pepperoni, etc.

Eggs. You should really be able to cook eggs. Eat the whole egg. Boiled, fried in butter or good oils, and scrambled are all good. My daughters are made out of eggs, butter and salt. If you're worried about cholesterol, stop it! I'll get back to the cholesterol issue in a bit. For now, eat as many eggs as you want.[61]

People can be dicks about eggs too. When it comes to weight loss just eat whatever eggs are best for your lifestyle. If you want to get fancy and eat cage free, free range eggs there are benefits like taste, better nutrient profile, better ethics about the treatment of animals, and more. I eat a brand called Happy Eggs. Don't let eating the best eggs be a barrier for you, eat whatever eggs you want. Keep your eyes on the prize not the tools.

Fat. Probably the least understood and most villainized food on the planet. Fat is essential. We would not be around as a species if it wasn't for fat in our diet. You can get your fat from both vegetable and animal sources. I have fat with every meal and sometimes just by itself. For our goal of weight loss, dietary fat will actually help mobilize body fat (specifically from the heart and liver), provide fuel for our brain and body in the form of ketones, and keep us from feeling hungry when we don't really need to eat. Fat makes most of our foods taste amazing. Foods that are marketed as "low fat" have the fat replaced with a ton of sugar just so you'll be able to eat it.
[62]

Trans fats or hydrogenated oils are really bad for you. In 2015 the FDA has mandated that they be removed from store shelves but they gave companies three years to do it. Don't eat fake butter and check labels for trans fats or hydrogenated vegetable oils. Margarine, packaged baked goods

---

[59] https://www.ncbi.nlm.nih.gov/pubmed/16500874
[60] https://www.ncbi.nlm.nih.gov/pmc/articles/PMC4772027/
[61] https://www.ncbi.nlm.nih.gov/pubmed/22037012
[62] https://www.ncbi.nlm.nih.gov/pmc/articles/PMC4245577/

and certain frying oils are the worst offenders. They will harden cell walls once they are endocytosed, leading to heart disease.[63]

Eat: Heavy cream, Cheese, Olive oil, Butter, Coconut oil, Almond oil, Lard, Walnuts, Macadamia, Peanuts, Cashews, Sour cream, Mayonnaise, Whole fat Greek yogurt, etc.

Add Ons. There are a few foods that you can include to spice things up (including spices!). Just be careful to look for sugars in the ingredients and avoid those (i.e. some ketchups). Here are some of the staples for everyone's diet: Coffee, Tea, Salt, Pepper, Cinnamon, Vinegar, Apple cider vinegar, Malt vinegar, Spices, Hot sauce, Ketchup, Mustard, Ranch dressing, Blue cheese dressing, Bone broth, etc.

Fast Food And Eating Out

Let's get something straight first, the goal is fat loss. If I wanted to create a model of human health I would not advise eating at fast food places but since most people reading this already do, we should address it. Remember, your fat loss is relative to where you're starting. If you routinely eat at these places, slightly changing what you order will have a tremendous impact on your weight. Fast food is especially appealing to people with limited time and/ or a limited budget and this program is for everyone so, don't be a snob.

Thanks to a growing low carb community there have been a ton of businesses ready to cash in on this market. Most restaurants have created low carb options instead of missing out on those sales. If you still want to eat at these places then stick to breadless/ sugarless/ potatoless menu items.

Here are a few of the most common restaurants and some of their less obesogenic options:

In-N-Out and Five Guys: Just order "protein style" and they'll serve you your burger in a lettuce wrap.

Fatburger: You can also get a lettuce wrapped burger here but they give you the option of having it in a tray as well as with a fried egg.

Jimmy John's: This sandwich shop offers an "Unwich" option. It's basically just any of their sandwiches wrapped in lettuce (ask for double wrapped to avoid a mess). Most sub shops can do this.

---

[63] http://www.cnn.com/2015/06/16/health/fda-trans-fat/index.html

Chipotle: Any of their bowls or salads without rice or tortillas (with double meat, sour cream and guacamole) are worth the trip.

Panera: The "Power Breakfast Egg Bowl with Steak" features 2 eggs, steak, tomatoes and avocados.

KFC: Grilled chicken is a slightly better option than breaded. Actually any unbreaded chicken including buffalo wings from a variety of places can keep you on track. Just make sure you're not getting them dipped in sugary sauces like teriyaki, stick to hot sauce or plain.

This is just a small sampling of the most popular offerings, with this in mind you can navigate just about anyone's menu and find a better option. You have to understand that this food is made with the cheapest possible ingredients to feed millions of people daily but because they are feeding millions of people this probably includes you or your kids, it is nice to know that by understanding the options you won't always have to avoid them to keep your insulin low. This is not the best case scenario but it doesn't have to be a death sentence for your weight loss.

Cheat Days

These are optional. Cheat days are basically just sugar and wheat days. They serve two purposes: greater compliance to the diet and increased leptin secretion. Whenever you lower your insulin for a few days you will have a corresponding drop in leptin levels. If you spike your insulin you will have a few hours that you can't access your fat stores but once insulin subsides you're left with elevated leptin levels. Your leptin levels will stay elevated for a few days, signalling your body to stop eating and start using energy (remember, what we are after is a spike in satiety hormones). Cheat days, when used correctly, can actually help us break through weight loss plateaus because of the corresponding leptin increase.[64]

If you follow the program correctly you will have an almost drug like response to cheat days. The first time you eat sugar or wheat on or after this program you will be inefficient at storing glucose. Your body will try to get rid of the excess sugar by raising your body temperature. You will also have a lower tolerance for the impending crash, not unlike a Thanksgiving day carb coma.

---

[64] https://www.ncbi.nlm.nih.gov/pmc/articles/PMC3602982/

What Not To Eat

Keep it simple. With the exception of cheat days, avoid refined foods. Powdered or liquified, sugar, corn, and wheat will lead to fat storage in your liver and eventually every other body part too. Essentially all refined starches are obesogenic, it doesn't matter what their source is. If it has been ground into a flour it may keep you from losing weight. As a species we have not developed hormones to stop over consumption of these ingredients. Your body does not have a built in limit for these hyper processed foods.

Try to stay away from artificial sweeteners. Artificial sweeteners still raise insulin regardless of their effect on blood glucose. Insulin drives weight gain.[65]

Until we fix the situation in your liver you will get greater results by avoiding additional insulin spiking foods like: white potatoes, white rice, and milk. If you are not insulin resistant these foods, in their natural state, will not lead to obesity.

Aside from fructose, another food that can trigger fat storage is beer. RNA (ribonucleic acid) degradation in yeast will lead to uric acid synthesis. This is also why people afflicted with gout arthritis should stay away from beer. High uric acid is the biggest contributor to triggering fat storage. Beer will trigger fat storage independent of fructose.[66][67]

---

[65] https://www.ncbi.nlm.nih.gov/pubmed/2887500
[66] https://www.ncbi.nlm.nih.gov/pubmed/16387838
[67] https://www.ncbi.nlm.nih.gov/pmc/articles/PMC1170497/

Section 4: Three week protocol

In this section we will go day by day for twenty-one days and highlight exactly what each day should look like. Follow along and you will not experience any hunger or a drop in energy but you will lose weight as fast as it is biologically possible.

Stay Focused

You have to keep your goal in mind to be able to shut out all the noise you're likely to hear when you start this program. The first priority of this program is for you to lose body fat. Nearly all of your health markers will improve when you drop excess fat but that is just an added benefit. What you're really after when you start this program is to see the scale move and your clothes get looser.

Getting Started

Pick a start date and an end date. Parkinson's law states that "Work expands to fill the time allotted for its completion". If you give yourself a year to lose five pounds it will take you a year to lose five pounds. If you give yourself a week it will take a week. If you don't have a deadline you won't have a sense of urgency.

Weigh yourself. The morning you start (and every morning after) you need to weigh yourself with minimal clothes on, after you pee, and before you drink anything. Try to eliminate variables like weighing yourself at different times so we can have a true comparison.

Take your before pictures. Front and side, full body and with good light. Keep in mind that you'll want to emulate these picture as close as possible when you take your after pictures (same lighting, angle, clothes, etc.). These are for your own benefit but if you'd like to share them with me I'd love to see them.

Take your measurements. Wrap a measuring tape around your waist at your belly button and record the measurement. You may also choose to measure your limbs and neck but I've found that the only number most people care about is the belly. Some personal trainers will measure everything and add all of them together so that the slightest change looks bigger than it actually is. This is for when your scale doesn't move and they need to keep you motivated. They'll say things like "You lost six total inches!" when in reality you are being measured slightly different every time and at every limb. Stick with measuring your waist at the belly button to avoid any bias or manipulation of numbers.

Get busy. Idle time is your enemy. If you get bored you will eat crappy food. Pick an activity that occupies your mind throughout the day. It can be work related, a sport, a charity or just get crazy about cleaning your house. Whatever you choose, if you're into it enough, food will never cross your mind.

Go shopping. Decide which meals you're likely to repeat and get a lot of those ingredients. Also, if you have a particular cookbook or recipe website you follow, get those ingredients. remember, you will run out of willpower sometimes so set yourself up for success by keeping your meal preparation easy and quick.

Daily Examples

The meals on these days are examples. You may choose to switch out which meats you like, which vegetables you prefer, and which spices you choose to flavor your food with. For example if it says chicken you can switch it to steak or ham. Only you will know which foods make you feel fuller for longer and that is our entire goal for eating. You'll probably find yourself eating only a few different things all of the time. What is important here is the time between meals.

It is important to overeat in the first week to avoid a sugar crash and really find out what makes you full and not want to eat. Think of your satiety hormones as a group of muscles that we have to strengthen. Likewise, your ability to fast needs to be built up slowly. Once you have control of your satiety hormones you may decide to try longer duration fasts.

The first week is designed to move you off of sugar. The second week is designed to increase the satiety effect of foods. Finally, the third week is all about fasting, fat loss, and autophagy. This should be surprisingly easy.

Day 1: Full feeding day

Breakfast: Scrambled eggs in butter with salt, bacon and coffee with heavy cream.
Lunch: Chipotle chicken bowl with sour cream and guacamole and beans. Iced tea.
Snacks whenever you want them: Apple, cheddar cheese, beef jerky, nuts

Dinner: Steak and broccoli with cheese sauce.

Day 2: Full feeding day

Breakfast: scrambled eggs with tomatillo salsa, sliced ham and coffee with heavy cream.
Lunch: two double doubles (protein style) from In-N-Out. Iced tea.
Snacks whenever you want them: pears, string cheese, hard boiled eggs with salt, nuts
Dinner: baked chicken, brussels sprouts with butter and salt.

Day 3: Full feeding day

Breakfast: spinach omelet with sour cream, coffee with heavy cream
Lunch: Fatburger with bacon and egg (protein style). Iced tea.
Snacks whenever you want them: pork rinds (chicharrones) with spinach dip
Dinner: pork chops and vegetable medley.
This is about the time that most of us experience sugar withdrawals. Keep some fruits around you all day.

Day 4: 16 hour fast

Breakfast: coffee with heavy cream.
Lunch: steak salad. Iced tea.
Snacks whenever you want them: raw vegetables with ranch dip.
Dinner: beef with broccoli.
You should be ready to skip breakfast at this point. You should not be waking up hungry.

Day 5: 16 hour fast

Breakfast: coffee with heavy cream.
Lunch: Jimmy John's Unwich. Iced tea.
Snacks whenever you want them: whole fat yogurt with fruit.
Dinner: steak and eggs with spinach, butter and salt.

Day 6: 16 hour fast

Breakfast: coffee with heavy cream.
Lunch: chicken wings (not breaded) with blue cheese. Iced tea.
Snacks whenever you want them: salad or fruit.

Dinner: stuffed bell peppers.

Day 7: 24 hour fast

Breakfast: coffee with heavy cream.
Lunch: Iced tea.
Dinner: spinach stuffed, bacon wrapped chicken breasts.

Day 8: 16 hour fast

Breakfast: coffee with heavy cream.
Lunch: taco salad (don't eat the tortilla). Iced tea.
Dinner: garlic lemon mahi mahi with green beans.

Day 9: 16 hour fast

Breakfast: coffee with heavy cream.
Lunch: green smoothie.
Dinner: shrimp stir fry.

Day 10: 36 hour fast

Fast as long as you can, try for 36 hours (last night's dinner to tomorrow's breakfast) If it's easy, skip tomorrow's breakfast. Drink only coffee with heavy cream and tea. It's important to remember that the longer you fast the quicker your liver will heal itself. Once your liver is back to a normal insulin sensitive state it will be really hard to gain any weight back.

Day 11: Full feeding day

Breakfast: scrambled eggs and sausage, coffee with heavy cream.
Lunch: steak salad.
Dinner: sloppy joe stuffed bell peppers.

Day 12: 16 hour fast

Breakfast: coffee with heavy cream.
Lunch: green smoothie.
Dinner: steak and broccoli with cheese.

Day 13: Cheat day (optional)

Breakfast: donuts, coffee with heavy cream.

Lunch: cheeseburger, fries and a milkshake.

Snacks whenever you want them: cookies, chips, chocolate

Dinner: pizza, ice cream

You will gain a few pounds after today but it typically disappears in 24 hours. If you've followed along perfectly the last two weeks, you will be groggy today and you will probably experience a rise in body temperature. You will, however, sleep like a baby.

Day 14: 24 hour fast

Breakfast: coffee with heavy cream.

Lunch: iced tea.

Dinner: pork chops and vegetable medley.

Day 15: 16 hour fast

Breakfast: coffee with heavy cream.

Lunch: green smoothie.

Dinner: ham and brussels sprouts with butter and salt.

Day 16: 16 hour fast

Breakfast: coffee with heavy cream.

Lunch: two protein style cheeseburgers. Iced tea.

Dinner: cobb salad.

Day 17: 16 hour fast

Breakfast: coffee with heavy cream.

Lunch: green smoothie.

Dinner: beef and broccoli stir fry.

Day 18: 16 hour fast

Breakfast: coffee with heavy cream.

Lunch: green smoothie.

Dinner: ahi steak with stir fry vegetables.

Day 19: Full feeding day

Breakfast: scrambled eggs with sour cream and avocado, bacon, and coffee with heavy cream.

Lunch: chipotle barbacoa bowl with guacamole and beans.

Dinner: garlic Greek chicken with asparagus.

Day 20: 24 hour fast

Breakfast: coffee with heavy cream.

Lunch: iced tea.

Dinner: pot roast and cauliflower with butter and salt.

Day 21: 36 hour fast

Fast as long as you can, try for 36 hours (last night's dinner to tomorrow's breakfast). If it's easy, skip tomorrow's breakfast.

Day 22: Conclusion

Weigh yourself, check your measurements and take your "after" pictures. Most people have a cheat day when they reach this point unless this is the day of the event you wanted to lose weight for. Depending on your starting weight you have likely lost twenty to thirty pounds and a myriad of health markers have probably improved. If you need to lose some more weight you should start over at day eight. This is how I regularly eat with some extended bouts of fasting (48 to 72 hours) mixed in once or twice a month.

Pro Tips

Pro tip: There are downstream effects on your tastebuds and sugar cravings caused by the bacteria in your mouth. When you have a sugar craving, try rinsing with mouthwash to reset your tastebuds and stop the cravings immediately. Plus, your breath can suffer when you are fasting or in ketosis. I just discovered this and it made my last three day fast effortless.

Pro tip: Stay busy. If you are not busy it can be extremely hard to fast or at least to not snack. When your mind is occupied eating can actually be an unwelcome interruption.

Pro tip: It's the consecutive hours fasted that gives us the hormonal response we are looking for. Interrupting your fast effectively resets the clock. If you don't feel good though, stop fasting.

Pro tip: Eat until you are full. We need that food to do its job, which is to keep our mind off of food for awhile.

Pro tip: Drink water. There is typically a lot of water in food, otherwise it would just be powder. When you are fasting you will need to drink a lot more water than you're used to. I've found mineral water helps me to retain water a little better so that I'm not peeing every five seconds.

Section 5: How exercise helps

You've likely heard that "abs are made in the kitchen" this is mostly true. The problem is that this insinuates that exercise doesn't aid in fat loss. When we are discussing the failed "energy balance theory" this is 100% correct, losing calories through exercise does not lead to fat loss. Although exercising to burn calories to lose fat doesn't work, exercising to create mitochondria and manipulate your body's resting metabolic rate to lose fat, does work. The fuel in your body can be used (by muscle) or stored (in fat). If we have more fat than muscle we will likely store more energy. If we have more muscle than fat our resting metabolic rate is higher and leads to greater energy expenditure and greater fat loss.[68]

The goal of this program is straight up fat loss so we will only deal with strategies that move us in that direction. If you don't currently exercise, pretty much anything you do will have a weight loss benefit. To lose fat you must be metabolically inefficient, this just means using more than the minimum effective dose of energy. Your body has to have a hard time keeping up. This means your exercise has to be a challenge, every time. People sometimes call this "muscle confusion" but whatever you want to call it you must make your body continually adapt. "Burning calories" by exercising is not a factor in weight loss but building muscle is.[69]

Resistance Training

All exercise comes down to squeezing and stretching muscles. When you work out you stretch a muscle then squeeze it tight, weights are just there to make the squeezing harder to do. Once you use up all of the fuel (glycogen) stored in those particular muscles, your muscles will start to take in more fuel (glucose, fatty acids, lactate) from the bloodstream leaving less blood glucose to be stored in your liver and fat cells. This can happen without insulin as resistance triggers glucose transporters (glut-4, glut-12).[70]

When you challenge yourself you will increase adrenaline and IGF-1 (insulin-like growth factor), both of which are highly catabolic to your fat tissue.[71] For a minimum effective dose of exercise you'll want to work the biggest muscle groups (back, legs, chest) to fatigue. If our only goal is fat loss that is all you need but some of us will want to work a particular muscle for

---

[68] https://www.ncbi.nlm.nih.gov/pubmed/19448716
[69] https://www.ncbi.nlm.nih.gov/pmc/articles/PMC2584808/
[70] https://www.ncbi.nlm.nih.gov/pubmed/9435517
[71] https://www.ncbi.nlm.nih.gov/pubmed/15831061

aesthetics, this isn't necessary but it is enjoyable (guys will want to do bicep curls, girls are mostly concerned about abs and butt). Resistance training will allow you to burn fat and build muscle at the same time as long as you challenge yourself every time and keep getting stronger.

Building muscle means creating more mitochondria (mitochondrial biogenesis), the more mitochondria you have the faster you will burn through your sugar and fat stores. Muscle is a much more metabolically active tissue than fat. Both fat and muscle want the fuel in your bloodstream so if you increase your muscle tissue you tip the scales in favor of fat burning versus fat storing.[72][73]

When you start lifting weights, think about your muscle tissue and your fat tissue as two cities with 1,000 residents each. It's your job to divide up the food for them so you split it 50/50. Over time some of the Fat town residents move away or die but a bunch of people moved into Muscleville. Obviously, you'll need to adjust your allocation. More and more of the food will go to the fine people of Muscleville as the population increases. Muscleville runs out of food everyday but the Fat town people don't even use their food, they just keep it stored away in case Muscleville gets hungry then they ship it over to them. At the end of the year Muscleville will have 5,000 people to feed and Fat town will have 200. Now how do you think your next meal will be divided up? More importantly, what is the obvious effect on your resting metabolic rate (RMR)? It goes up!

Running

Long slow cardio makes you better at long slow cardio, not fat loss. We adapt to become more efficient at utilizing fuel for any given exercise. Once we've adapted to the exercise we will become better at conserving our energy during that particular exercise. For fat loss we must remain inefficient. Long distance runners tend to shift their body composition to favor fat storage over time. If you choose the long slow cardio path, just make sure it stays a challenge, running up and down hills is a great tool for staying inefficient. Running the same three to five miles every week will soon lose it's effectiveness for fat loss. Women specifically will have a really hard time accessing most of their glycogen stores while running at a steady state.[74][75][76]

[72] http://www.cell.com/trends/endocrinology-metabolism/fulltext/S1043-2760(16)30109-6
[73] https://www.ncbi.nlm.nih.gov/pubmed/21817111
[74] http://www.dailymail.co.uk/sciencetech/article-3276926/The-pointlessness-long-distance-runner.html
[75] http://nymag.com/scienceofus/2015/10/on-the-mysteries-of-marathon-weight-gain.html
[76] https://www.ncbi.nlm.nih.gov/pubmed/2744924

Sprinting Or Interval Training

Beware of sprinting if you are not properly trained for it. Us common folk will get injured pretty quickly if we jump right into it. With that said; sprinting, resting, and sprinting some more is one of the most inefficient exercises and most potent for fat loss. Interval training tries to emulate this with spin classes, kettlebell workouts, group exercise programs, and bootcamps. Going all out, resting and repeating will enable you to tap into your fat stores faster than almost any other protocol.[77][78][79]

Swimming And Cold Exposure

By far the simplest exercise strategy for weight loss is swimming in water below eighty-degrees. As I've stated, remaining metabolically inefficient is the quickest path to fat loss. As a warm blooded animal there is no way to become metabolically efficient while constantly trying to keep your body's core temperature elevated in sub eighty-degree water. Your body will not stop trying to warm itself up so it will very quickly burn through it's glycogen stores and begin freeing up body fat for fuel. This why you are super hungry after a day at the beach or pool.[80][81][82]

How do we know when we are using fat as fuel instead of sugar? Easy, it's all in our breath. Scientists have observed that by measuring the carbon we breath out they can tell what we are using as fuel. This is called respiratory quotient or RQ value.

What is RQ value? The RQ is essentially the ratio of carbon dioxide eliminated to oxygen consumed. Roughly: RQ = C02 eliminated / O2 consumed. An RQ closer to 1 typically means more carbohydrate is being burned and a value closer to 0.7 typically means fat is being burned.

Sleep

The less you sleep, the more insulin resistant you are. Sleep plays a vital role in regulating metabolism. We've discussed that one of the mechanisms that keeps us fat is leptin resistance

[77] https://www.ncbi.nlm.nih.gov/pubmed/26243014
[78] https://www.nerdfitness.com/blog/cardio-vs-hiit-vs-weights-rebooting-our-research/
[79] https://www.ncbi.nlm.nih.gov/pubmed/25675374
[80] http://abcnews.go.com/Health/Wellness/nasa-scientist-chills-body-shed-pounds/story?id=12000983
[81] https://www.ncbi.nlm.nih.gov/pmc/articles/PMC3650516/
[82] https://www.ncbi.nlm.nih.gov/pubmed/2233284

and when we only have six hours of sleep or less we experience a 19% drop in leptin levels. You'll experience this with increased sugar cravings and drowsiness. In a recent study, healthy young men that slept just five hours per night for just one week experienced a 10% to 15% drop in testosterone levels leading to decreased libido, strength, focus, and increased insulin resistance and fatigue.[838485]

In my own experience, I have seen weight loss plateau when clients slept less than eight hours per night for a few nights in a row. Once they were able to get a full night's sleep (eight hours plus) their weight loss continued.

Conclusion

Whichever exercise program you choose to start just remember it has to be a challenge, every single time. Our bodies and brains are adapting non stop to our behaviors and environment. By adapting I mean, making it easier, once it becomes easy you will not benefit from it anymore. If you are clueless about what to do there are a ton of resources available to you. You could buy a couple of sessions from a trainer who looks like you want to look, join a group class, or you could check out the thousands of free programs and tutorials on YouTube (I still do this).

My favorite exercise program is without a doubt a solid kettlebell routine. A twenty or thirty pound kettlebell is relatively inexpensive at Walmart or on Craigslist and will last forever. So, a kettlebell and access to YouTube are more than you need for a total body workout that will sculpt your body, make you functionally strong, and kick your ass every-damn-time.

Shortly after the release of this manual I'll start work on my next project, which will focus solely on exercise. "Building Muscle For People In A Hurry".

Make sure that you are healthy enough to start an exercise regimen by talking with a medical doctor.

---

[83] https://www.ncbi.nlm.nih.gov/pmc/articles/PMC3767932/
[84] https://www.ncbi.nlm.nih.gov/pubmed/20371664
[85] http://www.cnn.com/2012/10/15/health/sleep-insulin-resistance/index.html

Section 6: Tools and resources

There are a couple of tools that can help you manage yourself on this program. There are apps that are specific to fasting, cook books that are dedicated to cooking without sugar and wheat, and even websites that hold you accountable to your commitments by letting you put your own money on the line and assigning a referee to make sure you're compliant. Some other resources include meal delivery services, low carb and ketogenic diet inspired snacks, online forums, and a community of people following this same program in a private group on Facebook.

One of my favorite ways to stick with something is to surround myself with it. So, while I'm fasting I'll listen to interviews with a scientist doing research in that field, read a book or research paper that matches the topic, or participate in online forums. Regardless of whether or not you use any of these resources your success will be directly related to how important the goal is to you. If losing fifty pounds is as important as breathing, then nothing can stop you, even without fancy apps or online support. With that said, here is a short list of some really cool products and services that can give you an advantage.

Apps

Zero. "Zero is a simple fasting tracker used for intermittent, circadian rhythm, and custom fasting. Choose your favorite fasting protocol and Zero will track your ongoing progress. Export your data to a spreadsheet for complete control."

Nom Nom Paleo. "The Nom Nom Paleo app makes food prep even more fun and inspirational, and takes all the guesswork out of cooking. And now that the Nom Nom Paleo app's available for both the iPhone and iPad, you can take these nomtastic recipes with you anywhere!"

mycircadianclock.org. "myCircadianClock helps you keep track of daily behaviors important for maintaining a healthy life, such as eating, sleeping, moving, and taking supplements and medications. Data that you share through the app as part of a research study will help researchers understand how daily timing of the behaviors influence health and wellbeing. At the same time, the app provides personalized insights into your daily rhythms"

Bit timer: "This app is designed for the no-frills, hard-core HIIT workout. This is the first interval timer you'll see with a set-up that is this fast and easy. Your workout should be intense, not your workout set up."

Websites

Unpaywall.org: "Officially launched on 4 April, Unpaywall is a free web-browser extension that hunts for papers in more than 5,300 repositories worldwide, including preprint servers and institutional databases."

Pubmed: "PubMed comprises over 26 million citations for biomedical literature from MEDLINE, life science journals, and online books. PubMed citations and abstracts include the fields of biomedicine and health, covering portions of the life sciences, behavioral sciences, chemical sciences, and bioengineering. PubMed also provides access to additional relevant web sites and links to the other NCBI molecular biology resources."

Google scholar: "Google Scholar allows you to search across a wide range of academic literature. It draws on information from journal publishers, university repositories, and other websites that it has identified as scholarly."

Edx.org: "edX is a massive open online course (MOOC) provider. It hosts online university-level courses in a wide range of disciplines to a worldwide student body, including some courses at no charge. It also conducts research into learning based on how people use its platform."

Foundmyfitness.com: "FoundMyFitness is Dr. Rhonda Patrick. Rhonda has extensive research experience in the fields of aging, cancer, nutrition. the platform by which Rhonda shares her insight from years of academic study and research on the best ways to increase healthspan."

Books

"Good calories, bad calories" by Gary Taubes

"Why we get fat" by Gary Taubes

"The case against sugar" by Gary Taubes

"The obesity code" by Jason Fung

"The complete guide to fasting" by Jason Fung and Jimmy Moore

"The big fat surprize" by Nina Teicholz
"Body by science" by Doug McGuff

"Keto Clarity" by Eric Westman and Jimmy Moore

"Tripping over the truth" by Travis Christofferson

"The fat switch" by Richard Johnson

"Bad science" by Ben Goldacre

"The great cholesterol myth" by Johnny Bowden and Stephen Sinatra

Products

23andme.com: Genetic testing for health and wellness reports.

Promethease.com: "Biomedical researchers, healthcare practitioners and customers of DNA testing services (such as 23andMe, Ancestry.com, FamilyTreeDNA, Genos, etc.) use Promethease to retrieve information published about their DNA variations. Most reports cost $5 and are produced in under 10 minutes. Much larger data files (such as imputed full genomes from dna.land) cost $10 and have increased runtime."

Ketonix.com: "Blood ketone measure requires test strips which are expensive and often require a prescription. Blood ketone measure sometimes fails and cost you twice, as you need to use another test strip. Blood ketone meter values differ between devices, even when it is the same model and brand."

Ketokookie.com: "Keto Kookie was created by two friends who went on a ketogenic diet and lost fat and felt amazing. But they had a hard time finding something sweet and ready made. So with health in mind, they invented Keto Kookie to make keto more fun, tasty, and convenient."

Section 7: Program Summary

For those of you that are really in a hurry and have skipped the entire manual, this is the section you came for. For everyone else, this is a useful reference while you're on this program.

The first step to take is to stop triggering weight gain by cutting out sugar, wheat, and beer. Basically, anything that spikes your insulin will make you gain weight. Then you need to give your liver a chance to fix itself, this is done through fasting induced autophagy. The problem is, fasting is extremely difficult if you are a "sugar burner". You will need to switch over to using fat as your primary fuel source to eliminate some of the side effects from fasting (mood swings, headaches). Now your focus should be on strengthening your satiety response to foods. At this point fasting should be effortless. Continue to eat foods with a high satiety response and space your meals out as far as you can. Balance fasting and feeding to stay healthy.

Section Summaries

Section one summary:

- Be skeptical and learn how to fact check people with science.
- You are different than everyone else. Because of your genetics, you will respond to food differently.
- If you start with a really crappy diet, a slightly less crappy diet will help you lose weight.
- Don't get technical. Call foods by their names (i.e. broccoli, steak) not categories (i.e. carbs, protein).
- The reason most diets work in the beginning is because they cut down on sugar.
- Most diets stop working because they only try to fix being fat not the reason you got fat. Also, they are too disruptive to your routine.
- Calorie decreases and increases happen at the same time as losing or gaining weight. They are not the cause.
- Hormones control your metabolism and most of your decisions.
- Some drugs can make you fat no matter what you eat or how much.

Section two summary:

- Fat gain can be triggered by fructose or beer. Once it is triggered foods that were fine before are now fattening to you.
- Once your liver becomes insulin resistant and fat, the rest of your body will follow.
- With a healthy liver most people are insulin sensitive and will stay lean.
- If you keep eating sugar and wheat you will become more and more insulin resistant and get fatter and fatter. You will eventually end up with type II diabetes.
- Cancer, heart disease, neurological disorders, depression, diabetes, obesity, arthritis, and many more problems can all be linked back to refined sugar consumption.
- 70% of chronic western diseases can be prevented or treated by eliminating high insulin levels caused by sugar and wheat consumption.
- Sometimes getting fat takes a very long time because your hormones are fighting against it as you mature. Conversely, sometimes children can become obese and get juvenile diabetes.
- There are extreme health consequences to weight gain that a lot of people won't experience until their late forties.

Section three summary:

- There are hormones that are designed to help you get rid of fat.
- You need to stop eating for some of these fat burning hormones to kick in.
- When you are fasting a lot of good things happen to your body, including fat loss.
- Autophagy is damage repair at the cellular level that only occurs while fasted.
- Autophagy helps to fight disease, clear away precancerous cells, and slows down the effects of aging on your organs.
- Autophagosomes are little organelles inside the cell. The more of these that are present the greater the reparative effects.
- If you fast for 24 hours you will experience a 300% rise in autophagosomes in the liver cells.
- Just as there are hormones that cause sugar cravings there are powerful hormones that tell you to stop eating. These hormones are the result of eating whole, unrefined foods.
- When you eat is at least as important as what you eat when it comes to weight loss. Space your meals for for greater weight loss. Balance feeding with fasting.

- Cheat days are not technically necessary but they can be beneficial. They can help with some hormone control and they can increase compliance to any eating plan.
- Unless it is cheat day, do not eat sugar, wheat, corn, potatoes, alcohol, milk.
- There are no natural satiety signal for refined foods. You will over eat these and they will not make you full.

Section four summary:

- The first week is designed to move you off of sugar. Eat a lot of foods the first week to help get off of sugar.
- Eat a lot of the same foods over and over for convenience.
- This is about the time that most of us experience sugar withdrawals. Keep some fruits around you all day.
- The second week is designed to increase the satiety effect of foods. Space your meals out into an intermittent fasting regimen.
- You should be ready to skip breakfast at this point. You should not be waking up hungry.
- The third week is all about fasting, fat loss, and autophagy. This should be surprisingly easy.
- There are some "pro tips" to help keep you on track throughout the program.

Section five summary:

- Lifting weights builds muscle and muscle will take a huge chunk of the fat and sugar out of your blood that would normally be used to make you fat.
- Long slow running will not lead to lasting weight loss.
- Once your body adapts to your exercise it will start to conserve energy while you do it, making it less effective for fat loss.
- If it is not a challenge to your body it will not change your body. You have to stay inefficient.
- Sprinting and interval training is the most effective for fat loss.
- Being cold makes your body constantly try to adapt by heating itself. You will burn through sugar stores very quickly and start using fat as fuel.
- Lack of sleep means lower testosterone, less willpower, higher insulin resistance, and slower weight loss.

Section six summary:

- There are apps that help you fast.
- There are websites dedicated to cooking without sugar and wheat.
- You should continue to learn about your body and health.
- If you surround yourself online and in person with information that reinforces what you're doing, you will have greater success.
- Check out www.weightlossforpeopleinahurry.com for more resources.

Giving Back

A portion of the proceeds from this book will go to Ketopet Sanctuary. To donate please visit www.ketopetsantuary.com

KetoPet Sanctuary

Human-Grade Cancer Therapy for Dogs

"Right now, on a 53-acre plot of land outside Austin, Texas, we at KetoPet Sanctuary (KPS) are doing something incredible. This isn't your typical canine rescue facility. KPS goes out of its way to rescue dogs with incurable, terminal cancer. Our goal isn't to provide hospice-like treatment for terminal dogs – of course we care for and love the animals, but instead of writing off the canine companions to their fate, we at KPS provide groundbreaking cancer therapy. We've been doing this since October of 2014 and the results are astounding. Plus, we guarantee each dog will have a loving forever home, for life"

Printed in Great Britain
by Amazon